DAIRY-FREE MEAL PREP

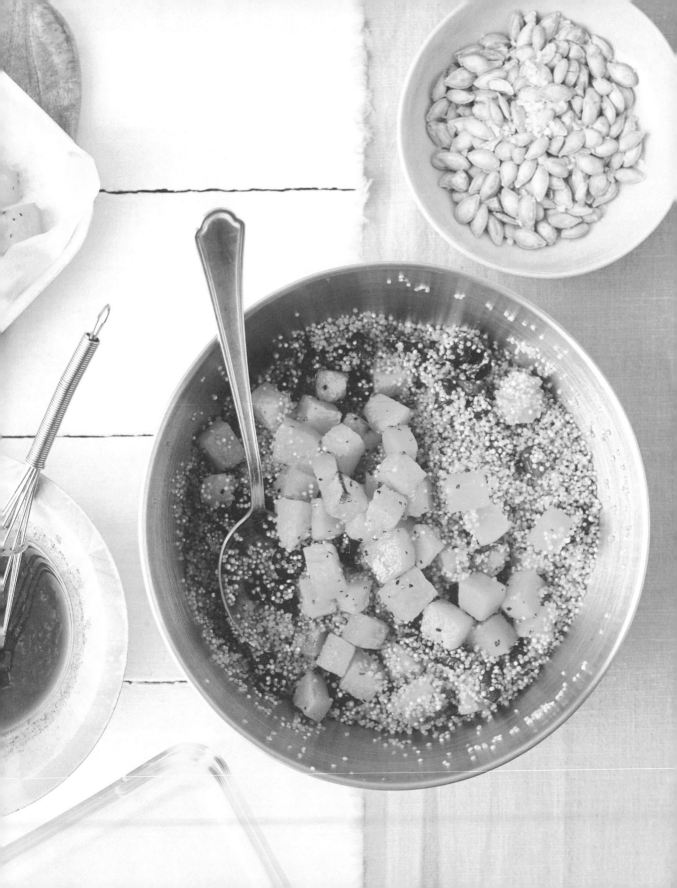

DAIRY-FREE
MEAL PREP

EASY, BUDGET-FRIENDLY MEALS
to COOK, PREP, GRAB, and GO

Silvana Nardone

PHOTOGRAPHY BY DARREN MUIR

ROCKRIDGE
PRESS

Interior and Cover Designer: Angie Chiu
Art Producer: Hannah Dickerson
Editor: Anna Pulley
Production Manager: Jose Olivera
Production Editor: Sigi Nacson

Photography © Darren Muir 2020
Author photo courtesy of Stephen Scott Gross

ISBN: Print 978-1-64739-259-8
Ebook 978-1-64739-260-4

R0

Boundless love to my beautiful children,
Isaiah and Chiara, my biggest supporters
both in and out of the kitchen.

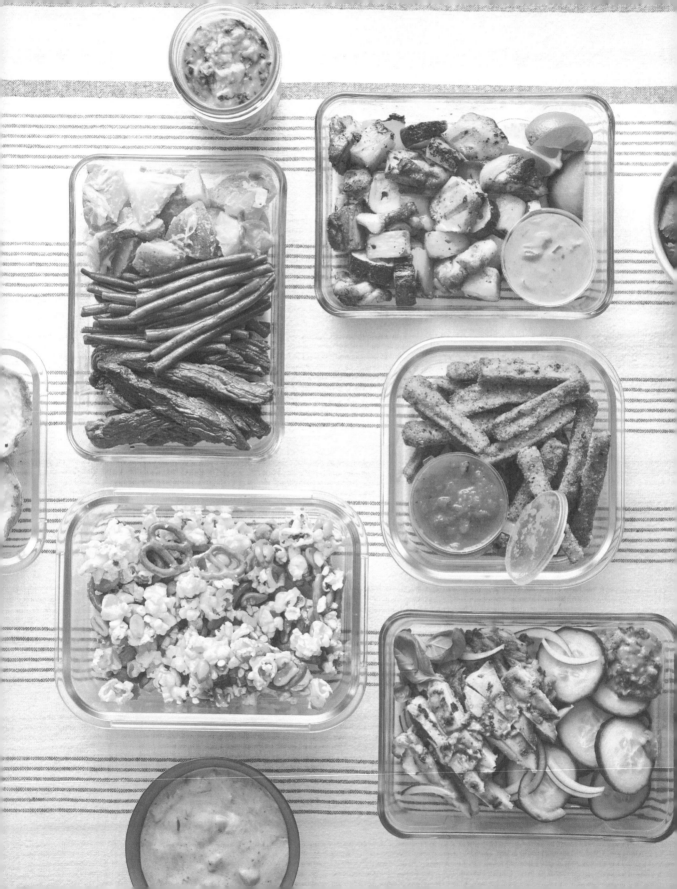

CONTENTS

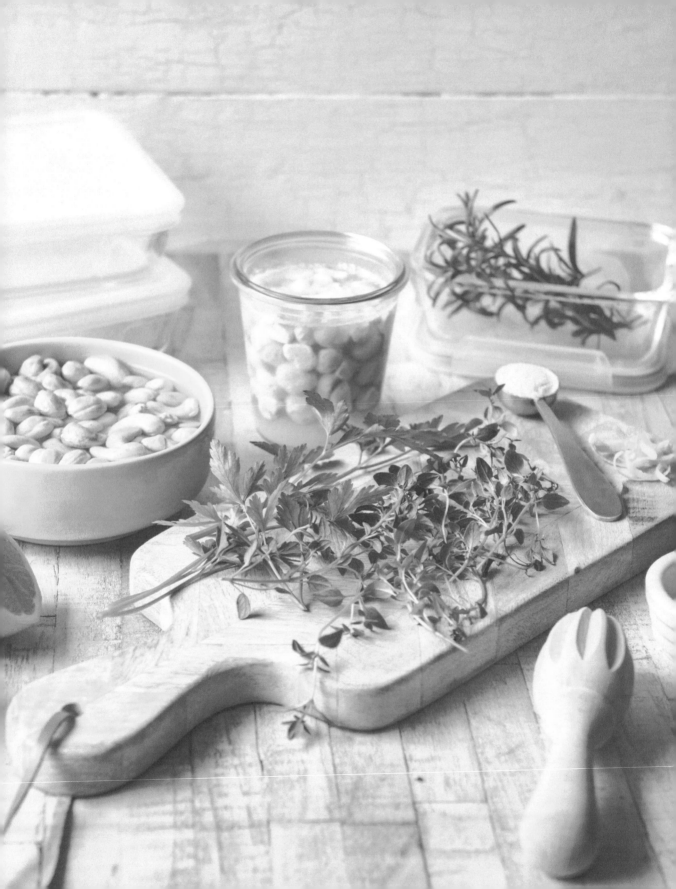

INTRODUCTION

My introduction to the dairy-free community was sudden. My then-10-year-old son, Isaiah, had been struggling with health issues, and I wouldn't stop digging until I figured out what the cause was—and how I could help him. Turns out, he was not only dairy intolerant, but also gluten intolerant. This was back when people didn't even know the word "gluten" and there were little to no dairy-free or gluten-free options at the health food store, let alone my local supermarket.

As a former bakery owner and food magazine editor, I knew I had the knowledge and experience to change that, not just for my family but also for anyone else who needed to cut dairy and gluten from his or her diet—for whatever reason. That's when I went into my kitchen and started playing around with different ingredients to create dairy-free and gluten-free versions of all the foods Isaiah loved. I failed time after time—until the day I didn't. Once I had cracked the code on how to re-create textures and flavors that were the same or better than the original, I knew I wanted to help other people cook and bake again.

Even with all my culinary experience, as a single mom raising two kids, I struggled to cook meals for my family. Having worked in commercial kitchens, I know that any prep is better than no prep, so I started doing meal prep at home. Doing meal prep not only ended my mealtime struggle, but also began saving me precious time and money. Deciding what meals to prep and in which order isn't exactly intuitive, though, and I want to show you how easy it can be to plan, cook, bake, and eat dairy-free.

The truth is that changing our dietary habits isn't easy. We get used to eating whatever we want, whenever we want. Luckily, that perspective shifts fast when you cut dairy from your diet and you suddenly feel energetic and lighter. You feel good. You feel like yourself. That changes everything.

Thank you for joining me on this dairy-free meal-prep journey. You're well on your way to eating healthier, spending less, and enjoying more time outside the kitchen with your family and friends.

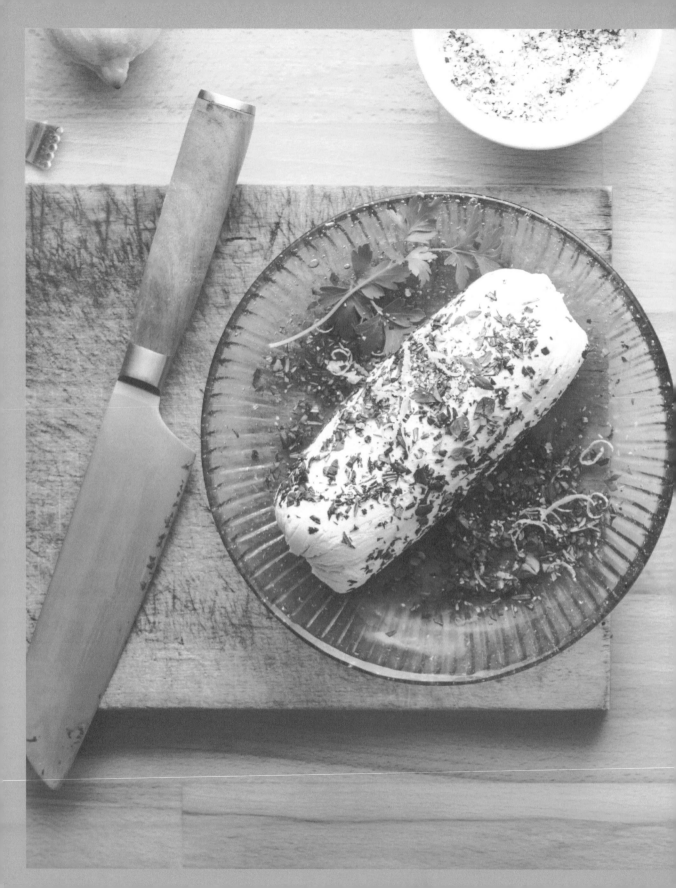

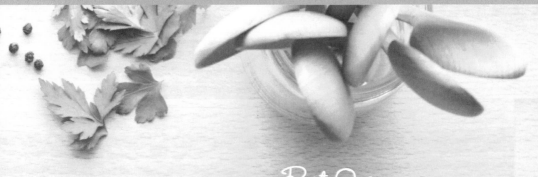

Part One

DAIRY-FREE MADE EASY

✖ ✖ ✖

Who among us have never asked ourselves the ongoing questions, "What am I going to make for breakfast?" "For lunch?" "For dinner?"

The reason I developed meal-prep recipes was partly in response to these questions. And believe me, you'll find plenty of answers in the recipes that follow—and even though they're all dairy-free, you won't feel like you're missing anything. The best part? When you meal prep for yourself or loved ones, you have an arsenal of recipes and dairy-free ingredients at your disposal for the week ahead.

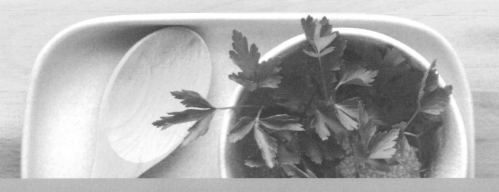

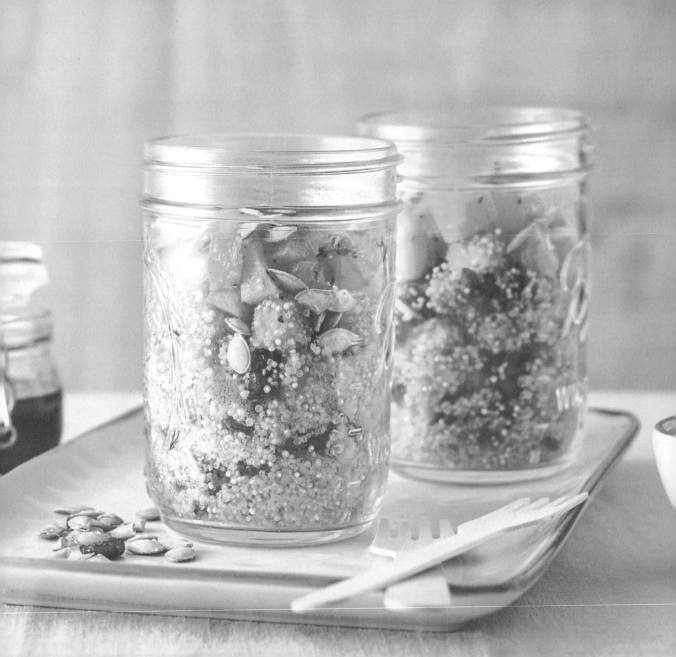

Quinoa Salad with
Butternut Squash and
Spiced Apple Cider Dressing
Page 52

Chapter One

WHY DAIRY-FREE?

✳ ✳ ✳

Before we start talking about meal prep, I'd like to address how dairy-free living may be intimidating at first. I'm here to tell you it doesn't have to be. Actually, cooking and baking dairy-free is easier than you think. When I first started on my dairy-free journey, in response to my son Isaiah's dairy-intolerance diagnosis, I was overwhelmed by the thought that we'd never again eat many meals we now took for granted, like Banana Pancake Muffin Tops (page 36) or Pressed Caesar Tuna Melts (page 131). Even bagels with cream cheese (see Dairy-Free Cream Cheese, page 101) or cereal with milk (see the dairy-free Cashew Milk, page 94) seemed like an impossibility.

Once you start feeling better—thanks to eliminating dairy from your diet—a mental shift happens and your food options widen. The first step is to remove all dairy—foods made from the milk of cows, goats, and sheep, and all its derivatives—from your kitchen. Then you replace your go-to ingredients with easy-to-make or store-bought dairy-free substitutes that you can eat and that look and taste like the originals. This will make going or staying dairy-free easier and make meal prep faster.

THE BEST THINGS IN LIFE ARE DAIRY-FREE

Whatever your reason for removing dairy from your life—whether you're allergic, intolerant, or want to improve your health—there are many benefits.

ANTI-AGING: Did you know that hormones found in dairy products can cause premature aging? Slowing the aging clock is just one long-term benefit of a dairy-free lifestyle.

CLEARER SKIN: If you get occasional breakouts, eczema, or rashes, eliminating dairy might make a difference in their frequency and severity. These skin conditions are the body's response to inflammation. Avoiding dairy altogether reduces the body's overall inflammation response, gives your skin a break, and can relieve other inflammation-related symptoms.

IMPROVED DIGESTION: People who have cut dairy from their diet attest that doing so can alleviate digestive issues such as acid reflux. Plus, if you're lactose intolerant and lack the proper enzymes needed to digest lactose—a natural sugar found in milk—having no dairy anymore means common indigestion symptoms such as bloating, gas, abdominal cramps, nausea, and diarrhea go away, too.

OVERALL WELL-BEING: Not eating dairy can result in increased energy levels, improved mood, and simply feeling better.

STRONGER IMMUNE SYSTEM: Because about 80 percent of our immune system is in the gut, anything that upsets the digestion—like dairy—could disrupt other systems in the body. Translation: Removing dairy from your diet can allow your immune system to get back to working properly.

THYROID HEALTH: Dairy products are mucus forming, and the protein in dairy has been found to increase inflammation in vital parts of the body, such as the thyroid gland and digestive tract. Since cutting out dairy, I've noticed improvements in my metabolism and energy levels, both of which can be linked to thyroid health.

4

THE DAIRY-FREE KITCHEN, SIMPLIFIED

Since beginning my family's dairy-free adventure, I've rebuilt my pantry by removing any foods containing dairy from the cabinets, fridge, and freezer in order to make space for new foods. The more recipe-ready you are before cooking and baking dairy-free, the more options you'll have for what you can make easily and quickly. Ultimately, all this comes down to feeling satisfied when it's time to sit down and enjoy a meal with your family and friends.

A DAIRY-FREE MEAL-PREP PANTRY

When I started meal prepping for my family, I refined my pantry so I could do more with less. I now stock my cabinets with essential ingredients that work well for meal prepping—meaning they're accessible, affordable, and store well—and that form the foundation for many meals I cook regularly. Then, I round out my kitchen options with what I refer to as flavor enhancers—ingredients that boost the flavor of almost everything. I suggest stocking the following staples to get your dairy-free meal-prep journey started.

BREAKFAST BASICS

- Almond butter
- Cinnamon, ground
- Flour, all-purpose or gluten-free
- Honey
- Maple syrup, pure
- Oats, old-fashioned rolled or certified gluten-free

FLAVOR ENHANCERS

- Broth, chicken or vegetable
- Chipotle paste
- Mustard, Dijon
- Tamari (gluten-free soy sauce)
- Tomato purée, canned

GRAINS AND BEANS

- Beans, black and cannellini, canned
- Quinoa, dried
- Rice, basmati
- Spaghetti or short-type pasta, dried

OILS, VINEGAR, AND SPICES

- Black pepper
- Chili powder
- Oil, avocado and olive
- Sea salt
- Vinegar, apple cider and rice wine

ROOTS AND TUBERS

- Garlic

- Onions, red and yellow
- Potatoes, Idaho and Yukon Gold

FOODS TO AVOID

When you eliminate dairy from your diet, some foods to avoid will be obvious to you, like milk and cheese, but others may be less so. Carefully read ingredient labels to avoid any hidden forms of dairy, such as casein or artificial or natural flavors that may be lurking in foods.

FOODS THAT DEFINITELY HAVE DAIRY

If a food's ingredient label includes any of the following, the food definitely contains dairy:

- Butter
- Buttermilk
- Cheese, including cream cheese and cottage cheese
- Cream of all types, including heavy and whipping
- Milk from cows, goats, and sheep, and condensed milk
- Sour cream
- Yogurt

FOODS THAT MAY HAVE DAIRY

This category of foods may not seem likely to include dairy. The reality is that packaged and processed foods like deli meats, salad dressings, chocolate, granola bars, hot dogs, potato chips,

protein powders, and spice blends can contain dairy. Food labels can be confusing, especially when you're new to dairy-free shopping. When in doubt, check the ingredient label for dairy or dairy by-products.

HIDDEN FORMS OF DAIRY IN INGREDIENT LISTS

There are two label terms to be aware of when buying packaged and processed foods: **non-dairy** and **dairy-free**. Contrary to popular belief, the term "non-dairy" does not actually mean milk-free.

The U.S. Food and Drug Administration's regulatory definition for non-dairy says that a product labeled as such can contain 0.5 percent or less milk by weight. The regulation allows for the presence of milk proteins, such as casein, whey, and other dairy derivatives. Casein is the main protein found in milk and cheese, and

6

whey, which is often used in protein powders, is the liquid part of milk that remains once the milk has been curdled and strained.

Carefully reading ingredient labels becomes critical, especially if you have a dairy allergy or your dairy intolerance is severe.

Some popular items that contain hidden dairy include artificial or natural flavorings, lactic acid starter culture, and prebiotics.

No regulatory definition exists for the term "dairy-free." However, this label is a better indicator of whether a food is actually free of dairy. Even better, thanks to the Food Allergen Labeling and Consumer Protection Act, food manufacturers are required to declare the top eight allergens, including dairy, on their labels. Look for the "contains milk" disclaimer below the ingredient list that states which allergen a product contains.

Another dietary label to look for is "vegan," which, based on dietary guidelines, means the product is dairy-free.

COMMON DAIRY SUBSTITUTIONS

The number of dairy-free products that now fill supermarket shelves, refrigerated cases, and freezer sections is incredible. You can either make dairy-free substitutions yourself or, for convenience, buy them at your local grocery store or online. When I don't have my homemade dairy-free basics on hand, these are my go-to store-bought dairy-free substitutions.

- **BUTTER:** For use in recipes and to spread on morning toast, I make my own Dairy-Free Butter (page 96). My preferred store brand is Miyoko's vegan butter, which is slightly salted and has a wonderfully emulsified, rich, spreadable texture.

- **CHEDDAR CHEESE:** I've taste-tested many shredded cheddar-style dairy-free cheeses, and my favorites are the Violife Just Like Cheddar Shreds and the Parmela Creamery Sharp Cheddar Meltable Shreds, which are aged for 30 days.

- **CHOCOLATE CHIPS:** It's not easy to find dairy-free chocolate chips. Even if you find semisweet chocolate chips without added milk, they might contain milk solids in the ingredient list. I've been using the dairy-free Enjoy Life Dark

Chocolate Morsels for more than a decade, and I recently discovered Hu Kitchen Snacking and Baking Dark Chocolate Gems, which are bigger in size for the serious chocolate lover.

- **CREAM:** I usually make this myself with cashews as the base (see Cashew Milk, page 94). If it is unsweetened, you can use it as a coffee creamer or as a substitute for heavy or whipping cream. When I buy it at the supermarket, I like Malk unsweetened oat and almond creamer or nutpods original unsweetened creamer, made with coconut cream and almonds.

- **MILK:** Cashew Milk (page 94) is the most neutral-tasting milk, which is why I use it in many recipes in this book. When I don't have it on hand, I like to buy Malk, which is ultra-creamy and less processed than most other dairy-free milks. If I want a neutral-flavored but naturally slightly sweeter flavor, I prefer Oatly!, which is made with oats. I always buy unsweetened so I can use the milk for both sweet and savory recipes.

· **MOZZARELLA:** After tasting a number of shredded mozzarella-style dairy-free cheeses, searching for great taste, texture, and meltability, I found two that meet my standards, and I regularly stock them in my fridge: the Violife cashew-based Just Like Mozzarella Shreds and the Parmela Creamery Meltable Mozzarella Shreds.

· **PARMESAN:** I make dairy-free Grated Parmesan Cheese (page 99) from pine nuts. When

I don't have any pine nuts in my fridge, I get Follow Your Heart parmesan-style cheese.

· **YOGURT:** Today's dairy-free yogurt options at the local grocery store are amazing in both flavor and texture. One of my favorite brands is Cocojune, a creamy, unsweetened coconut-based yogurt that's great for recipes. They also have fun, fruity flavors like strawberry-rhubarb and lemon-elderflower. Another favorite brand is Lavva, a zero-sugar-added yogurt made from pili nuts, which is wonderfully tart. I enjoy it on its own or in smoothies.

9

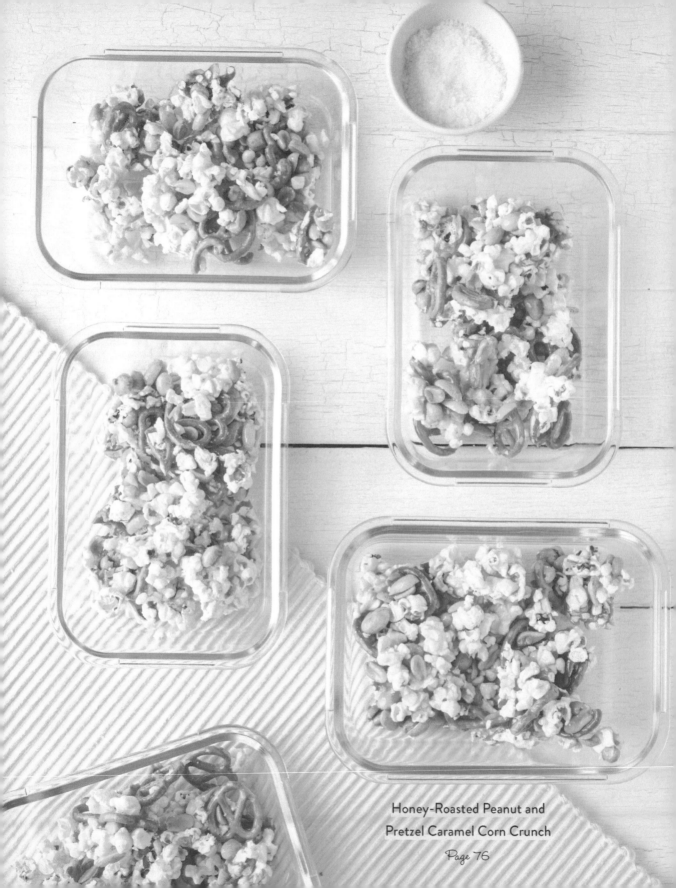

Honey-Roasted Peanut and
Pretzel Caramel Corn Crunch

Page 76

Chapter Two

WHY MEAL PREP?

❊ ❊ ❊

Think you don't have time to feed yourself or your family easy and delicious dairy-free meals during the week? Think again. Meal prepping is a small sacrifice of time with a huge payoff. Plus, learning the basic building blocks of meal prep means you can spend less time in the kitchen and more time doing what you love. Once you get the hang of meal prepping, it becomes easy to mix and match lunches and dinners to fit your dietary needs, or to plan meals based on what's in season. Among the many benefits you'll reap, you'll find that meal prepping saves time and money, helps with portion control, encourages consistent healthy eating—as with already prepped foods, there is no need for takeout—and reduces the overall stress that feeding yourself or your family can cause.

MEAL-PREP FUNDAMENTALS

Working in restaurant kitchens and owning my own bakery have taught me the fundamentals of being an efficient cook and baker—in use of time, energy, and money. What's the secret? It's easy: Prep and cook things days ahead and store them in the fridge or freezer for when they're needed. When it's time to eat, all you need to do is reheat and eat, or assemble and serve.

The basic prep tasks include washing and chopping fresh vegetables when you get home from the supermarket and batch-cooking some multi-use ingredients, such as quinoa, and ready-to-eat meals. Everything is then stored in reusable, portion-sized containers and is clearly labeled with masking tape so you can grab and go. And because you made it, you know exactly what's in it.

EASY DOES IT

When first starting to meal prep, go easy on yourself and coast into it with a few simple meals so you don't feel overwhelmed or get discouraged. I recommend mastering some staple recipes like Grated Parmesan Cheese (page 99), a simple topping for most comfort foods; White Cream Sauce (page 103) for favorites like Chicken and Broccoli Roll-Ups with Cheddar Cheese Dipping Sauce (page 31); and Baked Bacon, Egg, and Cheese Cups (page 27), a low-maintenance recipe for which your oven does all the work. When you're ready, you can add more variety with the bonus meal-prep recipes in part three of this cookbook, including riffs on restaurant favorites like Chicken Pasta with Creamy Vodka Sauce (page 143) or Spicy Sichuan Beef with Mixed Vegetables (page 142).

INGREDIENT MULTI-USE

I like to use certain ingredients in a couple of different ways among various recipes to save time and money, an approach that goes to the heart of meal prep. When you prep or cook, you can use one or two versatile ingredients— like chicken, potatoes, cauliflower, or rice—in other meals that go beyond the recipes listed for any given meal-prep week.

A BATCH MADE IN HEAVEN

There's added value in batch cooking a few meals at the same time, in a relatively short period. Whether it's breakfast, lunch, or dinner, you can sometimes save time and effort by focusing on making a couple of meals, storing them, and having them handy when you're experiencing the greatest time demands at home. Other times, you may not need to make your meals in advance.

START WITH A CLEAN SLATE

When you start with a clean kitchen, the meal prepping goes much faster. Add to that having lots of clean, uncluttered counter space (or even a dining table) and stacks of clean, empty storage containers, and you're well on your way to meal prepping with ease.

STICK WITH THE PLAN

Don't be tempted at the last minute to squeeze in an extra meal that's not on the week's menu. That can derail your essential tasks and slow you down, as well as cause unnecessary stress by requiring more food shopping, juggling of time, additional prepping and cooking, and, of course, cleanup.

What Not to Prep

Not everything lends itself to successful food storage. Foods that brown easily won't last out the week (think avocado, raw apples, or bananas, if not blended into a recipe). It's the same for foods that get soggy and greasy when reheated, such as fried foods and cream-based foods (dairy-free or not) that can separate when reheated.

13

STORAGE TIPS

The key to successful meal prep is properly storing the foods you prepare. You'll want to invest in resealable airtight containers. I prefer clear containers so I can easily see what's inside without opening them, as well as containers that nest so they don't take up a bunch of space in my fridge, cabinets, or freezer.

CONTAIN YOURSELF

So, how do you decide which containers are best for you? First, take a look at your (and your family's) lifestyle and eating habits. Do you eat breakfast on the go? Lunch in the office? Dinner as a family? Decide what containers make sense, starting with what the containers are made of (BPA-free plastic, glass, or metal), whether you need a leak-proof seal for transporting them, whether they need to have multiple compartments for various foods, or if they are microwave- and freezer-safe.

I prefer glass containers with locking lids, which are ideal for storing meals. With glass, you won't have to worry about food stains and smells left behind, and the containers are dishwasher safe, freezable, microwave safe, and oven safe. Translation: They can go from fridge to oven without the added step of transferring the contents to heatproof containers. Plus, with glass there's no worrying about possible chemicals leaching into the foods, as can happen with plastics. Having locking lids means you can take your meals on the go without the risk of leakage, and your food will stay fresher for longer.

Having containers in a variety of shapes and sizes is key for most lifestyles. If your family eats dinner together, using one large container to reheat the entire meal is more efficient, saves you time, frees up space in your fridge, and leaves you with less cleanup at the end of the meal.

If you take your lunch to go, glass can be heavy, however, and impractical to carry. Instead, look for BPA-free silicone collapsible food-storage containers. Expand the container to fill it, and when you're finished with your meal, just flatten the container to save space. What's another lunch option? Stainless-steel bento lunch boxes, which have multiple compartments to keep the parts of your meal separate.

To store your week's worth of meals, transfer the prepared foods to small, shallow containers and refrigerate them. For food safety reasons, hot foods can stay out for a maximum of two hours before they need refrigeration. Once packaged, foods should be stored only for as long as indicated in the recipes. See page 15 for a helpful chart with food storage guidelines.

LABEL WITH LOVE

Clearly label and organize the prepped recipes, especially ones that go in the freezer, so later on you can easily find what you're looking for. I like to include the name of the dish and the date I cooked it, so I know how long I have to eat what's inside the container.

	FRIDGE	FREEZER
Salads: egg salad, tuna salad, chicken salad, pasta salad	3 TO 5 DAYS	DOES NOT FREEZE WELL
Hamburger, meatloaf, and other dishes made with ground meat (raw)	1 TO 2 DAYS	3 TO 4 MONTHS
Steaks: beef, pork, lamb (raw)	3 TO 5 DAYS	3 TO 4 MONTHS
Chops: beef, pork, lamb (raw)	3 TO 5 DAYS	4 TO 6 MONTHS
Roasts: beef, pork, lamb (raw)	3 TO 5 DAYS	4 TO 12 MONTHS
Whole chicken or turkey (raw)	1 TO 2 DAYS	1 YEAR
Pieces: chicken or turkey (raw)	1 TO 2 DAYS	9 MONTHS
Soups and stews with vegetables and meat	3 TO 4 DAYS	2 TO 3 MONTHS
Pizza	3 TO 4 DAYS	1 TO 2 MONTHS
Beef, lamb, pork, or chicken (cooked)	3 TO 4 DAYS	2 TO 6 MONTHS

*Chart based on FoodSafety.gov

THAWING AND REHEATING

The meal prep recipes in this cookbook are intended to generate meals that will go in the fridge for the week or that can be frozen. Also, if you're feeling ambitious, you can make a double batch and freeze for later.

When thawing and reheating the foods, you'll see that some recipes can go straight from the freezer to the oven, while others are better if allowed to thaw overnight in the fridge before reheating and serving; I reference this in the recipes.

KITCHEN EQUIPMENT

Here are some kitchen tools that will help make meal prepping faster and easier. The truth is, you don't need anything out of the ordinary to meal prep, but when you're batch cooking or making dairy-free staples, you could definitely up your game with these trusty kitchen assistants.

MUST-HAVES

DUTCH OVEN: This versatile pot can go from stovetop to oven to fridge. It's my go-to cooking vessel for stews, soups, chilis, and braised meats.

8-INCH CHEF'S KNIFE: A versatile, sharp chef's knife helps you get the prep done fast.

12-INCH SKILLET: This skillet does all the heavy lifting for quick cooking.

CUTTING BOARD(S): A large cutting board makes prepping the veggies easier. There's plenty of room to chop up a bunch of carrots *and* a handful of onions for the week's recipes, for example. I prefer wooden cutting boards for general use and dishwasher-safe, BPA-free plastic cutting boards for meats.

LARGE SILICONE SPATULA: Wooden spoons have their place, but a silicone spatula is great for stirring and gets into saucepan corners easily.

MEASURING CUPS AND SPOONS: Measurement accuracy is important, especially when you're multitasking. It ensures that recipes turn out correctly, and it reduces and eliminates food waste. Also, if you're just starting to cook, measuring the ingredients for any recipe teaches you about portion sizes until you are comfortable enough to wing it or improvise.

ELECTRIC PRESSURE COOKER, SUCH AS THE INSTANT POT: Considered the ultimate meal-prepping appliance, the Instant Pot is a pressure cooker, slow cooker, rice cooker, steamer, yogurt maker, and egg cooker, all rolled into one. It's great for large-batch cooking and for sautéing, steaming, and warming foods.

HIGH-SPEED BLENDER: Simply put, high-speed blenders are more powerful than the average blender, which means you get a better, faster outcome for dairy-free milks and smoothies. You can also make a soup from raw to cooked in 5 minutes. Plus, when you're making dairy-free versions of base ingredients like milk or cheese, texture is everything. You'll save time, also, as you won't need a sieve to strain out the little pieces of ingredients that are left unprocessed by the average blender. The jars for blenders vary somewhat in size, from as small as 48 ounces to as large as 72 ounces. Be careful not to fill above the maximum line; if necessary, process recipes in two batches.

ABOUT MEAL PREP AND THE RECIPES

17

In part two, you'll find six weeks of meal preps and recipes that start easy and grow in complexity, beginning with just three recipes to make for the first two weeks and gradually progressing to five recipes per week, including breakfast, lunch, dinner, and snacks.

Each meal-prep plan makes enough servings to feed one person for five days. If you are feeding more than one person or you want leftovers, then double or triple the recipes accordingly.

Meal-prep weeks 1 and 2 (page 23): 1 breakfast, 2 lunches or dinners
Meal-prep weeks 3 and 4 (page 43): 1 breakfast, 3 lunches or dinners
Meal-prep weeks 5 and 6 (page 65): 1 breakfast, 3 lunches or dinners, 1 snack

In part three, you'll find more recipes that you can add to the weekly meal-prep plans in this book or mix-and-match to build your own weekly meal-prep plans. You'll also find my favorite DIY dairy-free staples that you can make at home so you have them ready to use.

All the recipes include tips like ingredient substitutions, information on how to store leftovers, and recipe variations, as well as nutritional information. They also have dietary labels for other allergens, such as Egg-Free, Gluten-Free, Nut-Free, and Vegetarian/Vegan. You'll also find some recipes labeled Gluten-Free Option, Nut-Free Option, or Soy-Free Option, which means they can be easily modified to accommodate these dietary restrictions.

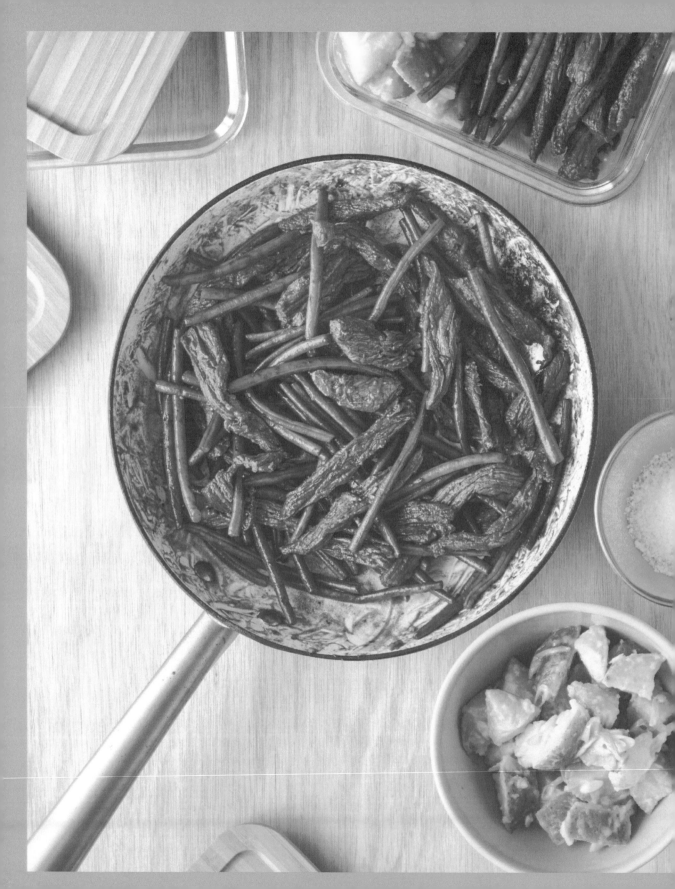

Part Two

DAIRY-FREE PREP AND RECIPES

❊ ❊ ❊

For the first couple of weeks, you'll start with a small number of recipes to ease into the meal-prep process, and along the way you'll pick up some great habits to make meal prepping a breeze. As you progress through this cookbook, the number of recipes for each week will increase from three to five. Note: Each meal prep is for one person, for weekday meals only. On weekends, you can enjoy trying out new recipes from part three of the cookbook or give yourself a break or dine out at your favorite local restaurant. Of course, depending on whether you are new to meal prepping or are a seasoned pro, you are always free to gauge your individual needs and make adjustments. Wherever you choose to begin the program, you'll find that all the meal preps provide the structure and support you'll need, with a focus on simple, doable, flavorful dairy-free recipes.

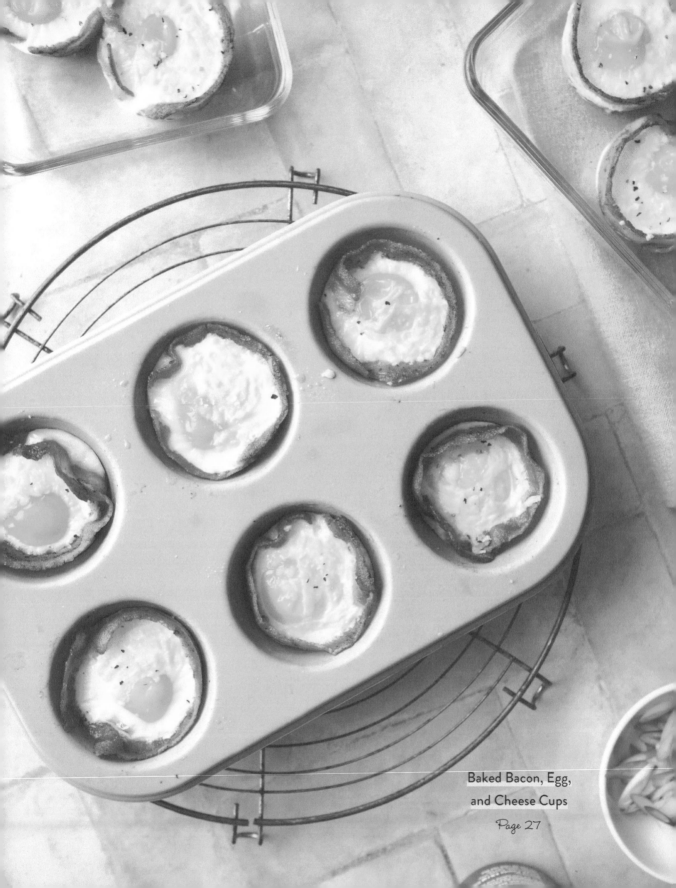

Baked Bacon, Egg,
and Cheese Cups

Page 27

Chapter Three

BEGINNERS' PREP, WEEKS 1 AND 2

❋ ❋ ❋

Welcome to the start of your dairy-free meal-prep journey! These recipes are low maintenance, meaning they don't require much hands-on, active prep time in the kitchen. You'll love the Baked Bacon, Egg, and Cheese Cups (page 27) for their simple assemble-and-bake technique, and the Tex-Mex Chili-'n'-Corn Veggie Mac (page 29), which is a one-pot meal that conveniently lasts all week long. Once you have your dairy-free pantry set up, you'll also notice that these recipes require only a quick trip to your local supermarket, because there's just a short grocery list of ingredients needed. You got this!

WEEK 1 RECIPES

Baked Bacon, Egg, and Cheese Cups

Tex-Mex Chili-'n'-Corn Veggie Mac

Chicken and Broccoli Roll-Ups with Cheddar Cheese
Dipping Sauce

WEEK 1 SHOPPING LIST

CANNED AND BOTTLED ITEMS

- ☐ Beans, black, 1 (15-ounce) can
- ☐ Tomatoes, crushed, 1 (28-ounce) can

DAIRY ALTERNATIVES AND EGGS

- ☐ Butter, Dairy-Free (page 96), or store-bought dairy-free (5 tablespoons)
- ☐ Cheese, dairy-free shredded cheddar-style (3½ cups plus 2 tablespoons)
- ☐ Cream Cheese, Dairy-Free (page 101), or store-bought plain dairy-free (1 cup)
- ☐ Eggs, large (10)
- ☐ Milk, Cashew (page 94), or unsweetened dairy-free (1 cup)

MEAT

- ☐ Bacon, sliced (8 ounces)
- ☐ Chicken, boneless, skinless breasts (1½ pounds)

PANTRY INGREDIENTS

- ☐ Bread crumbs or gluten-free rice cereal crumbs (1 cup)
- ☐ Chili powder
- ☐ Cooking spray, nonstick
- ☐ Cumin, ground
- ☐ Flour, all-purpose or gluten-free
- ☐ Oil, olive
- ☐ Pasta, short-type regular or gluten-free (8 ounces)
- ☐ Pepper, freshly ground black
- ☐ Salt

PRODUCE

- ☐ Bell pepper, any color (1)
- ☐ Broccoli, fresh (1 head, or 9 ounces)
- ☐ Carrot (1)
- ☐ Corn kernels, fresh or frozen (2 shucked ears or 1 [10-ounce] package frozen)
- ☐ Garlic (1 small head)

- ☐ Mushrooms, button,
  1 (10-ounce) package
- ☐ Onion (1)
- ☐ Scallions (1 bunch)

- ☐ Meat Mallet (optional)
- ☐ Toothpicks

WEEK 1 STEP-BY-STEP PREP

1. Preheat the oven to 375°F. Prep and bake the Baked Bacon, Egg, and Cheese Cups (page 27).

2. While the Baked Bacon, Egg, and Cheese Cups bake, make the dipping sauce on the stovetop for the Chicken and Broccoli Roll-Ups with Cheddar Cheese Dipping Sauce (page 31). Divide the prepared sauce between 2 small resealable containers and cover, label, and store in the fridge.

3. Prep the roll-ups for the Chicken and Broccoli Roll-Ups with Cheddar Cheese Dipping Sauce (page 31).

4. When the Baked Bacon, Egg, and Cheese Cups come out of the oven, bake the roll-ups, also at 375°F. Transfer the prepared egg cups to 5 medium resealable containers (2 per container). Cover, label, and store in the fridge.

5. While the roll-ups bake, prep and cook the Tex-Mex Chili-'n'-Corn Veggie Mac (page 29) on the stovetop. Divide the veggie mac among 3 medium resealable containers, topping each evenly with some cheese. Cover, label, and refrigerate.

6. Divide the chicken roll-ups among 4 medium resealable containers and cover, label, and store in the fridge.

25

WEEK 1 MEAL PLAN

	BREAKFAST	LUNCH/DINNER
DAY 1	Baked Bacon, Egg, and Cheese Cups	Tex-Mex Chili-'n'-Corn Veggie Mac
DAY 2	Baked Bacon, Egg, and Cheese Cups	Chicken and Broccoli Roll-Ups with Cheddar Cheese Dipping Sauce
DAY 3	Baked Bacon, Egg, and Cheese Cups	Tex-Mex Chili-'n'-Corn Veggie Mac
DAY 4	Baked Bacon, Egg, and Cheese Cups	Chicken and Broccoli Roll-Ups with Cheddar Cheese Dipping Sauce
DAY 5	Baked Bacon, Egg, and Cheese Cups	Tex-Mex Chili-'n'-Corn Veggie Mac

Baked Bacon, Egg, and Cheese Cups
Makes 10 egg cups

What's better than the diner classic that is the egg, bacon, and cheese sandwich? Maybe these cups. The best part is that these muffin-style breakfast cups are packed with protein and take only about 30 minutes to make. I always bake extra cups and freeze them for later. Serve these easy-to-prep breakfast cups with chopped scallions or minced fresh parsley, and for some heat, drizzle them with your favorite hot sauce.

PREP TIME: 10 minutes

COOK TIME: 24 minutes

Nonstick cooking spray
10 bacon slices
10 large eggs
½ cup plus 2 tablespoons shredded dairy-free cheddar-style cheese
Salt
Freshly ground black pepper

1. Preheat the oven to 375°F. Coat 10 cups of a standard muffin tin with cooking spray.

2. In a large skillet over medium heat, cook the bacon for 10 to 12 minutes, turning the slices once about halfway through, until crisp but still pliable. Transfer to paper towels to drain.

3. Line each muffin cup with 1 slice of bacon, starting on the bottom and bending it to line the inside of the cup.

4. Crack 1 egg into each muffin cup and top each egg with 1 tablespoon shredded cheese. Season with salt and pepper.

5. Bake for about 12 minutes, until the eggs are set. Gently remove the egg cups from the tin.

Continues →

27

STORAGE: Transfer the prepared egg cups to 5 medium resealable containers, placing 2 egg cups in each container. Cover, label, and refrigerate for up to 5 days, or freeze for up to 3 months.

REHEAT FROM THE FRIDGE: Bake the egg cups in a 350°F toaster oven for about 10 minutes or until warmed through and the bacon is crisp again. Or, place the egg cups on a microwave-safe plate and microwave on high power for about 30 seconds, until heated through.

REHEAT FROM THE FREEZER: Place the egg cups in the fridge overnight to thaw. Follow the above instructions for reheating from the fridge.

MIX IT UP: Swap in thin slices of Canadian bacon or ham for different protein options.

Per Serving (2 egg cups): Calories: 363; Total fat: 28g; Carbohydrates: 4g; Cholesterol: 414mg; Fiber: 0g; Protein: 27g; Sugar: 1g

Tex-Mex Chili-'n'-Corn Veggie Mac

Makes 3 servings

I love to make this veggie mac in summer when corn is in high season, but the truth is that if you use thawed frozen corn kernels, the recipe can be made mostly with pantry items, yielding a year-round meal-prep favorite for lunches and dinners.

PREP TIME: 15 minutes

COOK TIME: 20 minutes

2 tablespoons olive oil

1 (10-ounce) package sliced button mushrooms

1 bell pepper, any color, seeded and chopped

1 cup fresh corn kernels (from 1 large ear)

1 carrot, chopped

½ onion, chopped

2 garlic cloves, finely chopped

1 tablespoon regular or gluten-free chili powder

2 teaspoons ground cumin

1 teaspoon salt, plus more as needed

½ teaspoon freshly ground black pepper, plus more as needed

1 (28-ounce) can crushed tomatoes, with juice

1 (15-ounce) can regular or gluten-free black beans, drained and rinsed

8 ounces short-type regular pasta or gluten-free pasta

1 cup shredded dairy-free cheddar-style cheese

1 scallion, white and green parts finely chopped, for serving

1. In a large pot over medium heat, heat the olive oil. Add the mushrooms, bell pepper, corn, carrot, onion, garlic, chili powder, cumin, 1 teaspoon salt, and the pepper. Stir to combine. Cook for about 10 minutes, until the vegetables soften.

2. Stir in the tomatoes, beans, and pasta and bring the mixture to a boil. Cook for about 9 minutes, adding a little water as needed, until the pasta is al dente. Taste and season with salt and pepper as needed. Toss to coat the pasta with the sauce.

Continues →

29

STORAGE: Evenly divide the veggie mac among 3 medium resealable containers, topping each evenly with one-third of the cheese. Cover, label, and refrigerate for up to 5 days, or freeze for up to 1 month.

REHEAT FROM THE FRIDGE: Transfer the veggie mac to an oven-safe dish and cover the container with aluminum foil. Bake in a 400°F oven for about 15 minutes, until heated through and the cheese on top is melted. Or, place in a microwave-safe dish and microwave on high power for 1 to 2 minutes, until heated through. To serve, scatter the chopped scallion over the top.

REHEAT FROM THE FREEZER: To thaw, place the container in the fridge overnight. Follow the above instructions for reheating from the fridge.

MAKE IT EASIER: Prep the scallion ahead: Finely chop the scallion and store in a resealable container with a damp paper towel to preserve freshness until needed. Also, speed things up by swapping in frozen mixed vegetables for the corn and carrot.

Per Serving: Calories: 785; Total fat: 23g; Carbohydrates: 127g; Cholesterol: 0mg; Fiber: 23g; Protein: 24g; Sugar: 26g

Chicken and Broccoli Roll-Ups with Cheddar Cheese Dipping Sauce

Makes 4 roll-ups

I started making roll-ups for the family because the kids were getting bored with the same old chicken recipes. The cheesy dipping sauce—made with a creamy béchamel-style base—adds an extra layer of fun at the dinner table.

PREP TIME: 15 minutes

COOK TIME: 40 minutes

FOR THE DIPPING SAUCE

1 tablespoon Dairy-Free Butter (page 96) or store-bought dairy-free butter

1 tablespoon all-purpose flour or gluten-free flour

1 cup unsweetened Cashew Milk (page 94) or store-bought dairy-free milk, warmed, or more as needed

1 cup shredded dairy-free cheddar-style cheese, divided

Salt

FOR THE ROLL-UPS

Salt

1½ cups fresh broccoli florets

1 cup Dairy-Free Cream Cheese (page 101) or store-bought dairy-free cream cheese, at room temperature

1 cup shredded dairy-free cheddar-style cheese, divided

Freshly ground black pepper

4 boneless, skinless chicken breasts (1½ pounds total)

¼ cup Dairy-Free Butter (page 96) or store-bought dairy-free butter, melted

1 cup bread crumbs or gluten-free crushed rice cereal

TO MAKE THE DIPPING SAUCE

1. In a small saucepan over medium heat, melt the butter. Whisk in the flour and cook for 1 minute. Gradually whisk in the warmed milk. Cook, whisking, for about 6 minutes, until the mixture is steaming hot and thick.

2. Remove the pan from the heat and sprinkle in the cheese, stirring until melted. Season with salt.

TO MAKE THE ROLL-UPS

3. Prepare a bowl of ice water.

4. Bring a large pot of salted water to a boil over high heat. Add the broccoli and cook for 1 to 1½ minutes, until crisp-tender. Using a slotted spoon, transfer the broccoli to the ice water. Drain well. Let cool slightly, then finely chop.

5. Preheat the oven to 375°F. Line a baking sheet with parchment paper.

Continues →

31

6. In a medium bowl, stir together the broccoli, cream cheese, and shredded cheese. Season with salt and pepper.

7. Place a large piece of plastic wrap or parchment paper on a work surface and put the chicken on it. Cover with another piece of wrap. Using a meat mallet or other heavy object such as a rolling pin or cast-iron skillet, flatten each chicken breast to about ⅛-inch thickness. Remove the top piece of wrap. Season the chicken on both sides with salt and pepper.

8. Evenly divide the broccoli mixture among the chicken breasts, spreading it to cover them almost

to the edges. Roll up the breasts and secure with toothpicks if needed.

9. Pour the melted butter into a shallow bowl. Place the bread crumbs in another shallow bowl. Dip the rolled breasts into the butter, turning to coat completely, then roll the breasts in the bread crumbs to coat completely.

10. Place the coated chicken roll-ups seam-side down on the prepared baking sheet.

11. Bake for about 25 minutes, or until crisp, cooked through, and the juices run clear when pricked with a tester. Remove the toothpicks.

STORAGE: Divide the dipping sauce among 4 small resealable containers. Cover, label, and refrigerate for up to 5 days. Divide the roll-ups among 4 medium resealable containers. Cover, label, and refrigerate for up to 5 days.

REHEAT FROM THE FRIDGE: To reheat in the oven, transfer the roll-up to an oven-safe dish and cover the dish with aluminum foil. Bake at 400°F for 15 to 20 minutes, until heated through. Meanwhile, slowly reheat the dipping sauce in a saucepan over low heat, adding more milk, if needed, to thin the sauce to your desired consistency. In a microwave, heat the roll-up in a microwave-safe dish on high for 2 minutes, until heated through. Separately, reheat the dipping sauce in a microwave-safe bowl on high, stirring halfway through, about 1½ minutes total. Cut the roll-up crosswise into slices, and serve with the dipping sauce.

SUBSTITUTION TIP: Swap in your favorite veggies for the broccoli, such as cooked asparagus or even blanched and drained spinach.

Per Serving (1 roll-up with sauce): Calories: 703; Total fat: 45g; Carbohydrates: 30g; Cholesterol: 98mg; Fiber: 5g; Protein: 45g; Sugar: 5g

WEEK 2 RECIPES

Banana Pancake Muffin Tops

Supreme Pizza Pasta Bake

Oven-Fried Black Bean, Corn, and Cheddar Taquitos

WEEK 2 SHOPPING LIST

CANNED AND BOTTLED ITEMS
- ☐ Beans, black, 1 (15-ounce) can
- ☐ Salsa, fresh, 1 (15.5-ounce) jar
- ☐ Sauce, enchilada, 1 (8-ounce) can
- ☐ Sauce, pizza, 1 (15-ounce) can

DAIRY ALTERNATIVES AND EGGS
- ☐ Cheese, shredded dairy-free cheddar-style (1 cup)
- ☐ Cheese, shredded dairy-free mozzarella-style (¾ cup)
- ☐ Egg, large (1)

MEAT
- ☐ Pepperoni, sliced (2 ounces)
- ☐ Sausage, ground Italian sweet or hot (8 ounces)

PANTRY INGREDIENTS
- ☐ Baking powder
- ☐ Cinnamon, ground
- ☐ Cooking spray, nonstick
- ☐ Flour, all-purpose or gluten-free
- ☐ Oil, avocado (¾ cup)

- ☐ Pasta, short-type regular or gluten-free (6 ounces)
- ☐ Pepper, freshly ground black
- ☐ Salt
- ☐ Sugar
- ☐ Syrup, pure maple
- ☐ Vanilla extract

PRODUCE
- ☐ Avocado (1)
- ☐ Bananas, ripe (2)
- ☐ Basil (1 bunch)
- ☐ Bell pepper, any color (1)
- ☐ Corn kernels, fresh or frozen (2 shucked ears or 1 [10-ounce] package frozen)
- ☐ Garlic (1 small head)
- ☐ Onions, red (2)

OTHER
- ☐ Tortillas, corn or flour, 6 (6-inch)

SPECIAL EQUIPMENT
- ☐ Pastry brush
- ☐ Toothpicks

Continues →

WEEK 2 STEP-BY-STEP PREP

1. Preheat the oven to 350°F. Prep and bake the Banana Pancake Muffin Tops (page 36). Let cool completely. Place 2 muffin tops in each of 5 small resealable containers and cover, label, and refrigerate.

2. While the muffins bake, prep and cook the Supreme Pizza Pasta Bake (page 38) on the stovetop. Divide the pasta bake between 2 medium resealable containers. Cover, label, and refrigerate.

3. While the pasta bakes, prep the Oven-Fried Black Bean, Corn, and Cheddar Taquitos (page 40).

4. When the pasta is done, adjust the oven temperature to 375°F. Bake the Oven-Fried Black Bean, Corn, and Cheddar Taquitos (page 40). Divide the 6 taquitos among 3 medium resealable containers. Cover, label, and store them in the fridge.

WEEK 2 MEAL PLAN

	BREAKFAST	LUNCH/DINNER
DAY 1	Banana Pancake Muffin Tops	Oven-Fried Black Bean, Corn, and Cheddar Taquitos
DAY 2	Banana Pancake Muffin Tops	Supreme Pizza Pasta Bake
DAY 3	Banana Pancake Muffin Tops	Oven-Fried Black Bean, Corn, and Cheddar Taquitos
DAY 4	Banana Pancake Muffin Tops	Supreme Pizza Pasta Bake
DAY 5	Banana Pancake Muffin Tops	Oven-Fried Black Bean, Corn, and Cheddar Taquitos

Banana Pancake Muffin Tops

Makes 10 muffin tops

I haven't met a kid who doesn't love banana bread. This version bakes as muffin tops and yields a fun-filled handheld breakfast treat, inspired by our many morning trips to Panera before my family had to go dairy-free. Sometimes I throw ½ cup chopped walnuts into the batter for texture and a little extra protein.

PREP TIME: 10 minutes

COOK TIME: 14 minutes

Nonstick cooking spray

1½ cups all-purpose flour or
   gluten-free flour

2 teaspoons baking powder

1½ teaspoons ground cinnamon

½ teaspoon salt

1 large egg, at room temperature

¾ cup sugar

2 ripe bananas, mashed (about ¾ cup)

½ cup avocado oil

1 teaspoon vanilla extract

Pure maple syrup, warmed,
   for serving (optional)

36

1. Preheat the oven to 350°F. Coat 2 baking sheets with cooking spray or line them with parchment paper. Set aside.

2. In a large bowl, whisk the flour, baking powder, cinnamon, and salt to combine.

3. In a small bowl, whisk the egg, sugar, mashed bananas, avocado oil, and vanilla until blended. Add the wet ingredients to the flour mixture and stir to combine.

4. Using an ice cream scoop or ⅓-cup measure, place mounds of batter about 2 inches apart on the prepared baking sheets.

5. Bake for 12 to 14 minutes, until golden and a toothpick inserted into the center comes out clean.

STORAGE: Let cool completely. Place 2 muffin tops in 5 small resealable containers. Cover, label, and refrigerate for up to 5 days.

REHEAT FROM THE FRIDGE: In a toaster oven, place a muffin top on the rack and toast on the medium setting for about 2 minutes, until warmed through. Or, loosely wrap a muffin top in a paper towel and microwave on high power for about 30 seconds, until heated through. Serve with warmed maple syrup, if desired.

MIX IT UP: Chocolate lover? Sprinkle 1 teaspoon chocolate chips on top of each mound of batter before baking, for an extra kick of sweet.

Per Serving (1 muffin top): Calories: 247; Total fat: 12g; Carbohydrates: 34g; Cholesterol: 19mg; Fiber: 3g; Protein: 3g; Sugar: 18g

Supreme Pizza Pasta Bake

Makes 2 servings

One evening years ago, when I didn't have time to make my own pizza dough, I decided to put all the flavors of my family's favorite supreme pizza into a pasta dish. Now, we're still enjoying that delicious idea. Mix and match the "toppings" to fashion this pasta based on your family's favorite pizza. I use store-bought pizza sauce as a time-saver, but you can also use homemade sauce if you have some on hand.

PREP TIME: 10 minutes

COOK TIME: 25 minutes

Salt

6 ounces short-type regular pasta or gluten-free pasta

8 ounces ground Italian sweet sausage or hot sausage

½ bell pepper, any color, chopped

½ red onion, chopped

1 garlic clove, chopped

½ (15-ounce) can pizza sauce

¾ cup shredded dairy-free mozzarella-style cheese

6 pepperoni slices

Fresh torn basil leaves, for serving

1. Bring a medium pot of salted water to a boil over high heat. Add the pasta and cook according to package directions, until barely al dente, about 8 minutes. Drain.

2. In a large ovenproof skillet over medium-high heat, cook the sausage for about 5 minutes, breaking up the meat with a spoon, until browned.

3. Stir in the bell pepper, red onion, and garlic. Cook for about 5 minutes more, stirring occasionally, until the vegetables are softened.

4. Stir in the pizza sauce and simmer for 5 minutes. Stir in the cooked pasta, and top with the cheese and pepperoni.

38

STORAGE: Divide the pasta between 2 medium resealable containers. Cover, label, and refrigerate for up to 5 days, or freeze for up to 1 month.

REHEAT FROM THE FRIDGE: Transfer the pasta to an oven-safe dish, cover the dish with aluminum foil, and bake in a 400°F oven for about 20 minutes, until heated through. Remove from the oven and preheat the broiler. Brown the top of the pasta for about 3 minutes, until crisp. To reheat in the microwave, heat on a microwave-safe plate on high power for about 3 minutes, until warmed through. Serve with fresh basil sprinkled on top.

REHEAT FROM THE FREEZER: To thaw, place the container in the fridge overnight. Reheat as from the fridge.

SUBSTITUTION TIP: Love your pizza extra cheesy? Add shredded dairy-free cheddar-style cheese along with the mozzarella-style cheese.

Per Serving: Calories: 861; Total fat: 41g; Carbohydrates: 86g; Cholesterol: 103mg; Fiber: 12g; Protein: 54g; Sugar: 6g

Oven-Fried Black Bean, Corn, and Cheddar Taquitos

Makes 6 taquitos

I used to buy the taquitos that I found in the freezer section of my local supermarket. Then one day I decided to make them myself, and there's been no turning back. I prefer oven-frying the taquitos, which makes for easy cleanup and less mess, since the filling stays wrapped in the tortillas better.

PREP TIME: 10 minutes

COOK TIME: 35 minutes

Nonstick cooking spray

1 (15-ounce) can regular or gluten-free black beans, drained but not rinsed

1 cup fresh corn kernels (from 1 large ear)

1 cup canned enchilada sauce

½ small red onion, chopped

2 garlic cloves, finely chopped

Salt

6 (6-inch) corn or flour tortillas

1 cup shredded dairy-free cheddar-style cheese

Avocado oil, for brushing

1 avocado, halved, pitted, and cut into slices, for serving (optional)

Jarred salsa, for serving (optional)

1. Preheat the oven to 375°F. Line a baking sheet with aluminum foil and generously coat it with cooking spray.

2. In a small saucepan over medium-high heat, stir together the beans, corn, enchilada sauce, red onion, and garlic. Bring to a boil. Reduce the heat and simmer for 20 minutes. Season to taste with salt. Using a fork, crush the beans slightly to blend into the sauce.

3. Heat a large skillet over low heat. Soften each tortilla in the dry skillet by heating over medium heat for about 15 seconds per side.

4. Place the tortillas on a work surface and spread each with about 2 tablespoons of the bean mixture. Sprinkle each with about 2 tablespoons cheese, then roll up tight and secure with a toothpick, if needed. Place the filled tortillas

40

seam-side down in a single layer on the prepared baking sheet. Brush the tortillas with oil.

5. Bake for about 15 minutes, until crispy, turning occasionally. Remove the toothpicks.

STORAGE: Divide the taquitos among 3 medium resealable containers, 2 per container. Cover, label, and refrigerate for up to 5 days, or place the taquitos in freezer bags and freeze for up to 3 months.

REHEAT FROM THE FRIDGE: Place the taquitos in a single layer on a baking sheet, cover loosely with foil, and bake in a 350°F toaster oven or traditional oven for 10 to 15 minutes, until heated through and crispy. Or, loosely wrap the taquitos in paper towels and microwave on high power for about 1 minute, until heated through. Serve with the avocado and salsa, if desired.

REHEAT FROM THE FREEZER: To thaw, place the freezer bag in the fridge overnight. Reheat and serve as from the fridge.

MAKE IT EASIER: If you prefer, use your microwave in place of a dry skillet to soften the tortillas. Wrap the stack of tortillas in damp paper towels and microwave on high power for about 1 minute, until warm and pliable.

SUBSTITUTION TIP: If you don't have enchilada sauce handy, use tomato purée seasoned with some chili powder and cumin to taste.

Per Serving (2 taquitos): Calories: 477; Total fat: 24g; Carbohydrates: 58g; Cholesterol: 0mg; Fiber: 15g; Protein: 12g; Sugar: 1g

41

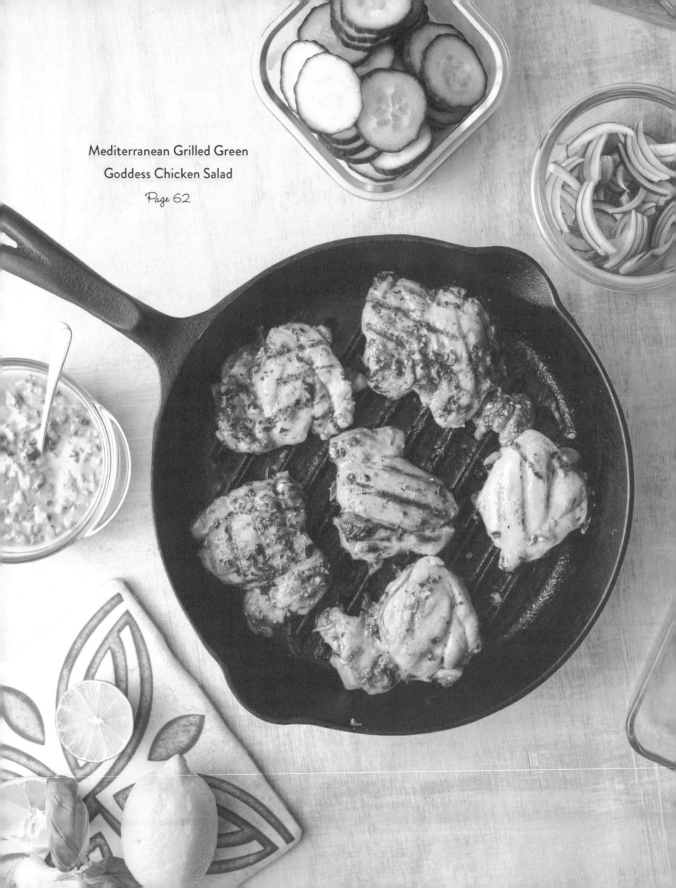

Mediterranean Grilled Green
Goddess Chicken Salad

Page 62

Chapter Four

YOU'RE REALLY COOKIN' NOW, WEEKS 3 AND 4

✻ ✻ ✻

Now you're ready to step up your meal-prep game by making one more meal this week, so schedule a little extra time for shopping and prepping. For these next two weeks, you'll be playing with classic recipes, like turning wonton soup into flavor-packed Wonton Burgers with Coleslaw (page 49) and apple pie into a fiber-packed, vitamin C–rich smoothie. You'll also be enjoying an easy Mediterranean grilled chicken salad smothered with creamy green goddess dressing, and will be virtually traveling to India with a recipe for Chicken Korma with Herbed Rice (page 58)—ready in a snap. If you're looking for a seasonal autumn salad that doubles as a Thanksgiving side dish, the Quinoa Salad with Butternut Squash and Spiced Apple Cider Dressing (page 52) will satisfy your comfort-food cravings.

WEEK 3 RECIPES

Apple Pie Smoothie

Wonton Burgers with Coleslaw

Spaghetti and Meatballs with Quick Creamed Spinach

Quinoa Salad with Butternut Squash and Spiced Apple Cider Dressing

WEEK 3 SHOPPING LIST

CANNED AND BOTTLED ITEMS
- ☐ Tomato purée, 1 (24-ounce) can

DAIRY ALTERNATIVES AND EGGS
- ☐ Cheese, Grated Parmesan (page 99), or store-bought dairy-free parmesan-style (¼ cup)
- ☐ Egg, large (1)
- ☐ Mayonnaise (2 tablespoons)
- ☐ Milk, Cashew (page 94), or store-bought unsweetened dairy-free (2 cups)
- ☐ Sour Cream, Dairy-Free (page 102), or store-bought dairy-free (½ cup)
- ☐ Yogurt, plain dairy-free (2½ cups)

MEAT
- ☐ Turkey, ground (1¾ pounds)

PANTRY INGREDIENTS
- ☐ Bread crumbs or gluten-free rice cereal crumbs (½ cup)

- ☐ Cayenne
- ☐ Cinnamon, ground
- ☐ Flour, all-purpose or gluten-free
- ☐ Nutmeg, ground
- ☐ Oats, certified gluten-free old-fashioned rolled (2½ cups)
- ☐ Oil, olive (¾ cup)
- ☐ Pepper, freshly ground black
- ☐ Quinoa (¾ cup)
- ☐ Salt
- ☐ Spaghetti (8 ounces)
- ☐ Sugar
- ☐ Syrup, date
- ☐ Syrup, pure maple
- ☐ Tamari
- ☐ Vanilla extract
- ☐ Vinegar, apple cider
- ☐ Vinegar, distilled white

PRODUCE
- ☐ Apples (5)
- ☐ Bananas (3)
- ☐ Basil (1 small bunch)

- ☐ Butternut squash, 1 small (12 ounces)
- ☐ Coleslaw mix, 1 (8-ounce) package
- ☐ Garlic (1 small head)
- ☐ Lemons (3)
- ☐ Onion (1)
- ☐ Parsley (1 small bunch)
- ☐ Scallions (1 small bunch)
- ☐ Spinach, frozen chopped, 1 (16-ounce) package

OTHER
- ☐ Burger buns (3)
- ☐ Cranberries, dried (3 tablespoons)
- ☐ Miso, dairy-free chickpea (1 teaspoon)
- ☐ Nutritional yeast (¼ cup)
- ☐ Probiotic powder, dairy-free
- ☐ Pumpkin seeds, roasted salted

SPECIAL EQUIPMENT
- ☐ Blender, high-speed

WEEK 3 STEP-BY-STEP PREP

1. If using, make the Cashew Milk (page 94) for the Spaghetti and Meatballs with Quick Creamed Spinach (page 50). Refrigerate in an airtight container.

2. Prep and cook the White Cream Sauce (page 103) on the stovetop for the Spaghetti and Meatballs with Quick Creamed Spinach (page 50). Cover, label, and refrigerate.

3. If using, make the Grated Parmesan Cheese (page 99) for the Spaghetti and Meatballs with Quick Creamed Spinach (page 50). Refrigerate in an airtight container.

4. If using, make the Dairy-Free Sour Cream (page 102) for the Spaghetti and Meatballs with Quick Creamed Spinach (page 50) and refrigerate in an airtight container.

5. Prep the Apple Pie Smoothies (page 48). Divide the baked apples among 5 medium resealable bags. To each bag, add ½ banana, 1 cup ice cubes, ½ cup oats, ¼ cup yogurt, and ½ teaspoon vanilla. Seal, label, and freeze the smoothie bags.

6. Preheat the oven to 400°F. Prep and bake the meatballs for the Spaghetti and Meatballs with Quick Creamed Spinach (page 50).

7. While the meatballs bake, prep and cook the creamed spinach. Let the creamed spinach cool slightly, then transfer to 4 small resealable containers and sprinkle with parmesan. Cover, label, and refrigerate.

Continues →

45

8. Cook the spaghetti for the Spaghetti and Meatballs with Quick Creamed Spinach (page 50). Drain.

9. Make the tomato sauce for the Spaghetti and Meatballs with Quick Creamed Spinach (page 50). Add the meatballs and cooked spaghetti. Let cool, then place the spaghetti and meatballs in 4 medium resealable containers; cover, label, and refrigerate.

10. Prep and mix the coleslaw and cook the burgers for the Wonton Burgers with Coleslaw (page 49).

Evenly divide the coleslaw among 3 small resealable containers. Cover, label, and refrigerate for up to 5 days. Let the burgers cool slightly, then place each one in a resealable bag. Label and refrigerate.

11. Prep and make the Quinoa Salad with Butternut Squash and Spiced Apple Cider Dressing (page 52). Transfer the quinoa salad to 3 medium resealable containers; label and refrigerate.

46

WEEK 3 MEAL PLAN

	BREAKFAST	LUNCH	DINNER
DAY 1	Apple Pie Smoothie	Spaghetti and Meatballs with Quick Creamed Spinach	Wonton Burgers with Coleslaw
DAY 2	Apple Pie Smoothie	Quinoa Salad with Butternut Squash and Spiced Apple Cider Dressing	Spaghetti and Meatballs with Quick Creamed Spinach
DAY 3	Apple Pie Smoothie	Spaghetti and Meatballs with Quick Creamed Spinach	Wonton Burgers with Coleslaw
DAY 4	Apple Pie Smoothie	Quinoa Salad with Butternut Squash and Spiced Apple Cider Dressing	Spaghetti and Meatballs with Quick Creamed Spinach
DAY 5	Apple Pie Smoothie	Wonton Burgers with Coleslaw	Quinoa Salad with Butternut Squash and Spiced Apple Cider Dressing

Apple Pie Smoothie

Makes 5 smoothies

This smoothie will make you think you're eating apple pie—no joke!
Plus, by prepping in advance, all you need to do is throw each
portion into the blender and you have breakfast in no time.
I like to use dairy-free yogurt to increase the protein
content and for its healthy probiotics.

PREP TIME: 10 minutes

COOK TIME: 10 minutes

5 apples, cored and chopped

2 tablespoons plus 1½ teaspoons sugar
    (optional)

2½ teaspoons ground cinnamon

2½ ripe bananas, halved

5 cups ice cubes

2½ cups certified gluten-free
    old-fashioned rolled oats

1¼ cups plain dairy-free yogurt

2½ teaspoons vanilla extract

1. Preheat the oven to 400°F.
   Line a baking sheet with parchment paper.

2. On the prepared baking sheet,
   toss together the apples, sugar
   (if using), and cinnamon. Spread
   the apples out in the pan.

3. Bake for about 10 minutes, until
   the apples are softened. Let cool.

STORAGE: Divide the apples evenly among 5 resealable freezer bags. In each bag, place
½ banana, 1 cup ice cubes, ½ cup oats, and ½ teaspoon vanilla. Seal the bags, label, and freeze
the apple mixture in the freezer for up to 1 month. Place ¼ cup yogurt in each of 5 small
resealable containers. Cover, label, and refrigerate the yogurt for up to 5 days.

TO SERVE: Transfer the contents of 1 frozen apple bag to a high-speed blender and add the
contents of 1 yogurt bag. Blend on high speed for about 3 minutes, until smooth and creamy,
adding a little water (1 tablespoon at a time) to thin the mix if necessary.

MIX IT UP: For more apple flavor, swap in ice cubes made from apple juice for the regular
ice cubes.

Per Serving (1 smoothie): Calories: 377; Total fat: 5g; Carbohydrates: 78g; Cholesterol: 0mg; Fiber: 12g; Protein: 9g;
Sugar: 35g

Wonton Burgers with Coleslaw

Makes 3 burgers

These burgers have the filling you'd find in a typical wonton soup, minus the wrapper—a fun flavor play on the classic Chinese starter, and the perfect meal for lunch or dinner. I use ground turkey in this recipe, but for a more traditional wonton flavor, use ground pork.

PREP TIME: 10 minutes

COOK TIME: 10 minutes

12 ounces ground turkey

1½ scallions, green and white parts finely chopped

1½ garlic cloves, finely chopped

3 teaspoons tamari, divided

¼ teaspoon salt, plus more for seasoning

¼ teaspoon freshly ground black pepper, plus more for seasoning

1½ tablespoons olive oil

1½ cups fresh coleslaw mix

1½ teaspoons apple cider vinegar

2 tablespoons mayonnaise

3 regular burger buns or gluten-free buns, split in half, for serving

1. In a medium bowl, mix the ground turkey, scallions, garlic, 2¼ teaspoons of the tamari, the salt, and pepper. Form the mixture into 3 patties.

2. In a large skillet over medium heat, heat the olive oil. Add the burgers and cook for about 4 minutes per side, turning once, until cooked through and no longer pink (they will feel firm).

3. In a medium bowl, toss together the coleslaw mix, vinegar, and remaining ¾ teaspoon tamari. Season to taste with salt and pepper.

49

STORAGE: Let the burgers cool slightly, then place each in a resealable bag. Seal, label, and refrigerate for up to 5 days. Divide the coleslaw among 3 small resealable containers. Cover, label, and refrigerate for up to 5 days.

REHEAT FROM THE FRIDGE: Place the burgers on a wire rack in a baking sheet. Warm in a 400°F oven for 3 to 5 minutes, until heated through. To reheat in the microwave, wrap the cooked burger in a damp paper towel and cook on low power for about 2 minutes, until heated through. To serve, spread 2 teaspoons mayonnaise on the bun bottom, then top each with a burger, add one-third of the slaw, and finish with the bun top.

MIX IT UP: For extra flavor, stir 1 teaspoon toasted sesame oil into the ground turkey mixture. Want some heat? Stir sriracha to taste into the mayonnaise before spreading on the burgers.

Per Serving (1 burger): Calories 412; Total fat 22g; Carbohydrates 28g; Cholesterol 93mg; Fiber 2g; Protein 26g; Sugar 6g

Spaghetti and Meatballs with Quick Creamed Spinach

Makes 4 servings

I love this cheesy creamed spinach, which is made in a flash by using a béchamel-type sauce, then stirring in dairy-free sour cream to deliver that classic flavor. The meatballs are light and airy, not dense and hard, thanks to the dairy-free milk.

PREP TIME: 15 minutes

COOK TIME: 35 minutes

Salt

8 ounces regular spaghetti or gluten-free

1 cup White Cream Sauce (page 103)

¼ cup Grated Parmesan Cheese (page 99) or store-bought dairy-free grated parmesan-style cheese, plus more for serving

½ cup Dairy-Free Sour Cream (page 102) or store-bought dairy-free sour cream

1 (16-ounce) package frozen chopped spinach, thawed and squeezed dry

Freshly ground black pepper

1 pound ground turkey

1 onion, finely chopped

2 garlic cloves, 1 finely chopped and 1 smashed

½ cup bread crumbs or crushed gluten-free rice cereal

½ cup Cashew Milk (page 94) or store-bought dairy-free milk

1 large egg

2 tablespoons chopped fresh parsley

1 tablespoon olive oil

1 (24-ounce) can tomato purée

8 fresh basil leaves

50

1. Bring a medium pot of salted water to a boil over high heat. Add the spaghetti and cook according to the package directions, until barely al dente. Drain.

2. Preheat the oven to 400°F. Line a baking sheet with parchment paper.

3. In a small saucepan over low heat, warm the white sauce for 2 minutes, stirring constantly, until heated through. Remove from the heat and stir in the parmesan until melted. Stir in the sour cream, then add the spinach and stir to combine. Season to taste with salt and pepper.

4. In a large bowl, mix the turkey, onion, chopped garlic, bread crumbs, milk, egg, parsley, and 1 teaspoon salt. Shape the mixture into 16 balls that are 1 inch in diameter, and place them on the prepared baking sheet.

5. Bake for 15 to 20 minutes, until the meatballs are cooked through.

6. In a large saucepan over medium heat, heat the olive oil. Add the smashed garlic and cook for about 2 minutes, until golden. Stir in the tomato purée and bring the sauce to a simmer, stirring occasionally.

7. Submerge the meatballs in the sauce, and return the sauce to a simmer. Cover the pan and cook for 20 minutes, stirring occasionally. Season to taste with about 1 teaspoon salt. Add the spaghetti, stir well, and heat until the pasta is warmed through and coated with the sauce.

STORAGE: Let the spaghetti and meatballs cool slightly. Meanwhile, transfer the creamed spinach to 4 small resealable containers and sprinkle with some parmesan. Cover, label, and refrigerate for up to 5 days. Place the spaghetti and meatballs in 4 medium resealable containers. Cover, label, and refrigerate for up to 5 days.

REHEAT FROM THE FRIDGE: Transfer the creamed spinach to an oven-safe dish, cover the dish with aluminum foil, and bake in a 400°F oven for about 15 minutes, until heated through. Transfer the spaghetti and meatballs also to an oven-safe dish, cover, and bake in the 400°F oven also for about 15 minutes, until heated through. To reheat in the microwave, transfer the spaghetti and meatballs to a microwave-safe dish and add 2 tablespoons water. Set a microwave-safe lid askew. Microwave on high power in 90-second intervals, stirring between each interval, until warmed through, about 6 minutes. Similarly, transfer the creamed spinach to a microwave-safe dish and add 1 tablespoon water. Set a microwave-safe lid askew. Also microwave on high power in 90-second intervals, stirring between each interval, until warmed through, about 3 minutes.

SUBSTITUTION TIP: For a more classic creamed spinach flavor, add ½ teaspoon Worcestershire sauce to the white cream sauce. If you're gluten-free, use gluten-free Worcestershire sauce.

Per Serving: Calories 585; Total fat 23g; Carbohydrates 59g; Cholesterol 141mg; Fiber 6g; Protein 37g; Sugar 10g

Quinoa Salad with Butternut Squash and Spiced Apple Cider Dressing

Makes 3 servings

This salad is perfect as a light meal, and it celebrates the flavors of fall with squash, apple cider, and cinnamon. I also like to multiply the recipe and serve it as a side dish at Thanksgiving or other fall gatherings.

PREP TIME: 10 minutes

COOK TIME: 30 minutes

1 small butternut squash (about 12 ounces), peeled, seeded, and cut into ½-inch cubes (about 3 cups)

3 tablespoons olive oil, divided

Salt

Freshly ground black pepper

¾ cup quinoa, rinsed well and drained

3 tablespoons dried cranberries

1½ tablespoons apple cider vinegar

1½ tablespoons pure maple syrup

¼ teaspoon cayenne pepper

Pinch of ground cinnamon

Roasted salted pumpkin seeds, for topping

1. Preheat the oven to 400°F.

2. Spread the squash cubes on a baking sheet and toss with 1½ tablespoons of the olive oil. Generously season with salt and pepper.

3. Roast for about 15 minutes, turning the cubes once halfway through the cooking time, until they are golden and tender.

4. In a saucepan over high heat, bring 1½ cups of salted water to a boil. Add the quinoa and cranberries. Cover the pan and simmer the quinoa for 15 minutes, until cooked through and the water has evaporated. Fluff with a fork, then transfer to a large bowl.

5. Meanwhile, in a small bowl, whisk together the vinegar, maple syrup, cayenne, and cinnamon. In a slow, steady stream, whisk in the

remaining 1½ tablespoons olive oil until blended and emulsified. Season to taste with salt and pepper.

6. To the quinoa in the bowl, add the roasted squash, the pumpkin seeds, and enough dressing to moisten the quinoa, reserving the remaining dressing for serving.

STORAGE: Transfer the quinoa salad to 3 medium resealable containers. Cover, label, and refrigerate for up to 5 days. Place the remaining dressing in a container to have handy.

TO SERVE FROM THE FRIDGE: Fluff the salad with a fork, and, if necessary, season again to taste with salt and pepper. Sprinkle on the remaining dressing.

MIX IT UP: For a summery version of this dish, swap in cubed fresh tomatoes, grilled corn kernels, and diced red onion, and use the herb-flecked Green Goddess Dressing (page 105) to serve.

Per Serving: Calories: 383; Total fat: 17g; Carbohydrates: 54g; Cholesterol: 0mg; Fiber: 6g; Protein: 7g; Sugar: 14g

WEEK 4 RECIPES

Banana, Maple, and Almond Butter Chia Pudding

Chicken Korma with Herbed Rice

Individual Cheeseburger Meatloaf with Quick-Pickled Veggies

Mediterranean Grilled Green Goddess Chicken Salad

WEEK 4 SHOPPING LIST

DAIRY ALTERNATIVES AND EGGS

- ☐ Almond butter, unsalted (2 tablespoons)
- ☐ Cheese, dairy-free cheddar-style (5 ounces)
- ☐ Coconut milk, canned (1¼ cups)
- ☐ Egg, large (1)
- ☐ Yogurt, plain dairy-free (1 cup)

MEAT

- ☐ Beef, ground (12 ounces)
- ☐ Chicken, boneless, skinless thighs (2½ pounds)

PANTRY INGREDIENTS

- ☐ Bread crumbs or gluten-free rice cereal crumbs (6 tablespoons)
- ☐ Chia seeds (½ cup)
- ☐ Cooking spray, nonstick
- ☐ Cumin, ground
- ☐ Ketchup (6 tablespoons)
- ☐ Oil, olive

- ☐ Pepper, freshly ground black
- ☐ Rice, basmati (1 cup)
- ☐ Salt
- ☐ Sugar
- ☐ Syrup, pure maple
- ☐ Vanilla extract
- ☐ Vinegar, apple cider (1 cup)

PRODUCE

- ☐ Banana (1)
- ☐ Basil (2 bunches)
- ☐ Bell pepper, red (2)
- ☐ Carrots (3)
- ☐ Cilantro (1 bunch)
- ☐ Cucumber (2)
- ☐ English cucumber (1)
- ☐ Garlic (1 head)
- ☐ Ginger (1-inch piece)
- ☐ Mint (1 bunch)
- ☐ Onions, red (4)
- ☐ Onions, white (2)

SPECIAL EQUIPMENT
- ☐ Basting brush
- ☐ Blender, high-speed
- ☐ Meat mallet (optional)
- ☐ Mini loaf pans (3)

WEEK 4 STEP-BY-STEP PREP

1. Make the Green Goddess Dressing (page 105) for the Mediterranean Grilled Green Goddess Chicken Salad (page 62). Refrigerate the dressing in an airtight container.

2. Preheat the oven to 350°F. Make and bake the meatloaves for the Individual Cheeseburger Meatloaf with Quick-Pickled Veggies (page 60). Let the mini meatloaves cool slightly, then transfer to 3 medium resealable containers. Cover, label, and store in the fridge.

3. Make the pickled veggies for the Individual Cheeseburger Meatloaf with Quick-Pickled Veggies (page 60). Divide the pickled vegetables among 3 small resealable bags, seal, label, and refrigerate.

4. Preheat a grill or grill pan to medium heat. Prep and cook the chicken for the Mediterranean Grilled Green Goddess Chicken Salad (page 62). Place the chicken in 3 medium resealable containers. Cover, label, and refrigerate.

5. Prep the red onion and cucumber for the Mediterranean Grilled Green Goddess Chicken Salad (page 62). Divide the red onion among 3 small resealable bags. Divide the cucumber among 3 small resealable bags. Seal the bags, label, and refrigerate.

6. Prep and cook the Chicken Korma with Herbed Rice (page 58) on the stovetop. Divide the chicken korma among 4 medium resealable containers and cover, label, and place in the fridge. Divide the rice among 4 small resealable containers and cover, label, and refrigerate. Divide the cilantro among 4 small resealable bags. Seal, label, and refrigerate.

7. Make the Banana, Maple, and Almond Butter Chia Pudding (page 57). Divide the chia pudding among 5 small resealable containers. Cover, label, and refrigerate.

WEEK 4 MEAL PLAN

	BREAKFAST	LUNCH	DINNER
DAY 1	Banana, Maple, and Almond Butter Chia Pudding	Chicken Korma with Herbed Rice	Individual Cheeseburger Meatloaf with Quick-Pickled Veggies
DAY 2	Banana, Maple, and Almond Butter Chia Pudding	Mediterranean Grilled Green Goddess Chicken Salad	Chicken Korma with Herbed Rice
DAY 3	Banana, Maple, and Almond Butter Chia Pudding	Individual Cheeseburger Meatloaf with Quick-Pickled Veggies	Mediterranean Grilled Green Goddess Chicken Salad
DAY 4	Banana, Maple, and Almond Butter Chia Pudding	Chicken Korma with Herbed Rice	Individual Cheeseburger Meatloaf with Quick-Pickled Veggies
DAY 5	Banana, Maple, and Almond Butter Chia Pudding	Chicken Korma with Herbed Rice	Mediterranean Grilled Green Goddess Chicken Salad

Banana, Maple, and Almond Butter Chia Pudding

Makes 5 puddings

I developed this make-ahead breakfast for two reasons: It's fast and easy to prep in advance, and it makes me feel good every time I eat it. The coconut milk and banana make it extra creamy.

PREP TIME: 10 minutes

1¼ cups canned coconut milk, well stirred
1¼ cups water
2 tablespoons unsalted almond butter
½ banana
1 tablespoon pure maple syrup
1 tablespoon vanilla extract
½ cup chia seeds

In a blender, combine the coconut milk, water, almond butter, banana, maple syrup, and vanilla. Blend on high speed until combined. Transfer to a medium bowl, stir in the chia seeds, and refrigerate for about 30 minutes, until thickened.

> **STORAGE:** Divide the chia pudding among 5 small resealable containers. Cover, label, and refrigerate for up to 5 days.
>
> **SUBSTITUTION TIP:** Not a fan of coconut? Swap in your favorite unsweetened dairy-free milk for the coconut milk.

Per Serving: Calories: 360; Total fat: 28g; Carbohydrates: 23g; Cholesterol: 0mg; Fiber: 11g; Protein: 8g; Sugar: 6g

57

Chicken Korma with Herbed Rice

Makes 4 servings

I developed this dish over the years by regularly eating two of my favorite types of cuisine—Indian and Mexican. Every time I eat at an Indian restaurant, I order chicken korma—chicken braised in a creamy sauce of yogurt and spices. The herbed rice was inspired by a dish I enjoyed at a Mexican restaurant, where I just had to ask the waiter for the recipe.

PREP TIME: 20 minutes

COOK TIME: 1 hour, 10 minutes

1¾ cups plus 3 tablespoons water, divided

¼ cup coarsely chopped white onion

3 garlic cloves, 1 smashed and 2 chopped

½ cup chopped fresh cilantro, divided, plus more for serving

Salt

2 tablespoons olive oil, divided

1 cup basmati rice, rinsed and drained

1½ pounds boneless, skinless chicken thighs, cut into chunks

Freshly ground black pepper

1 red onion, sliced

1 (1-inch) piece fresh ginger, peeled and sliced

2 teaspoons ground cumin

1 cup plain dairy-free yogurt

1. In a blender, combine 1¾ cups of the water, the white onion, smashed garlic, ¼ cup of the cilantro, and 1 teaspoon salt. Blend until smooth.

2. In a 2-quart saucepan with a tight-fitting lid, set over medium heat, heat 1 tablespoon of the olive oil.

3. Add the rice and stir to coat. Cook for 5 minutes. Add the onion mixture and bring the rice to a boil. Cook for about 10 minutes, until the liquid is reduced by half. Turn the heat to low and cover the pan; cook for about 10 minutes more, until the rice is tender and the liquid is absorbed. Turn off the heat and let sit, covered, for 15 minutes. Fluff the rice with a fork.

4. Season the chicken all over with salt and pepper.

58

5. In a large skillet over medium heat, heat the remaining tablespoon olive oil. Add the chicken and cook for 8 minutes, or until golden. Remove the chicken from the skillet.

6. Add the red onion and ginger to the skillet and cook for about 5 minutes, until softened.

7. Stir in the chopped garlic and the cumin. Cook for about 3 minutes, until fragrant.

8. Place the chicken back into the skillet and stir in the yogurt and remaining 3 tablespoons water. Taste and season with salt. Turn the heat to low and simmer for about 8 minutes, until heated through.

STORAGE: Divide the chicken korma among 4 medium resealable containers. Cover, label, and refrigerate for up to 3 days, or freeze for up to 1 month. Divide the rice among 4 small resealable containers. Cover, label, and refrigerate for up to 4 days, or freeze for up to 1 month. Divide the remaining ¼ cup cilantro among 4 small resealable bags. Seal, label, and refrigerate for up to 3 days.

REHEAT FROM THE FRIDGE: In a skillet over medium heat, cook the chicken for about 5 minutes, until warmed through. Or, place the chicken on a microwave-safe plate, cover with a microwave-safe lid set askew, and microwave on high power for about 3 minutes. When reheating, add water if needed, 1 tablespoon at a time.

Transfer the rice to a microwave-safe dish, and add 1 tablespoon water. Using a fork, break up any clumps of rice and cover with a microwave-safe lid or a damp paper towel. Microwave on high power for about 1 minute, fluffing with a fork halfway through, until the rice is heated through. To serve, top the rice with the chicken and sprinkle with the cilantro.

REHEAT FROM THE FREEZER: To thaw, place the chicken and rice containers in the fridge overnight. Follow the reheating and serving as from the fridge.

SUBSTITUTION TIP: For more authentic flavor, stir 1 teaspoon garam masala into the sauce in step 7. If you prefer, use chicken breasts in place of the thighs. For a nutty crunch, top with chopped roasted cashews before serving.

Per Serving: Calories 463 Total fat 15g Carbohydrates 42g Cholesterol 143mg Fiber 2g Protein 36g Sugar 1g

Individual Cheeseburger Meatloaf with Quick-Pickled Veggies

Makes 3 mini meatloaves

This recipe has all the makings of a classic cheeseburger, but it's in the shape of a mini meatloaf. Instead of making one big meatloaf, these single-serving loaves make it easier to meal prep for the week—and the meat stays nice and moist with all the juices locked inside.

PREP TIME: 15 minutes, plus 10 minutes to pickle

COOK TIME: 40 minutes

¾ cup apple cider vinegar

1½ tablespoons sugar

1½ cups thinly sliced vegetables, such as carrot, radish, red onion, bell pepper, and cucumber

Nonstick cooking spray

2 teaspoons olive oil

½ onion, chopped

1 carrot, grated

1 garlic clove, grated

12 ounces ground beef

6 tablespoons ketchup, divided

1 large egg, lightly beaten

¼ cup plus 2 tablespoons bread crumbs or crushed gluten-free rice cereal

5 ounces dairy-free cheddar-style cheese, 3 ounces cut into cubes, the rest shredded (½ cup)

Salt

Freshly ground black pepper

1. In a medium resealable container, whisk the vinegar and sugar until dissolved. Add the sliced vegetables, stir to combine, and let sit for at least 10 minutes, until pickled.

2. Preheat the oven to 350°F. Coat 3 mini loaf pans with cooking spray.

3. In a skillet over medium heat, heat the olive oil. Add the chopped onion and carrot. Cook for about 5 minutes, until softened. Stir in the garlic and cook for about 1 minute more. Let cool.

4. In a medium bowl, mix the ground beef, 3 tablespoons of the ketchup, the egg, bread crumbs, the onion mixture from the skillet, the cheddar cheese cubes, ¾ teaspoon salt, and ¾ teaspoon pepper. Divide the meatloaf mixture evenly

among the prepared loaf pans, rounding the tops. Spread each meatloaf with 1 tablespoon of the remaining ketchup.

5. Bake for about 30 minutes, until cooked through.

STORAGE: Let the mini meatloaves cool slightly, then transfer to 3 medium resealable containers. Cover, label, and refrigerate for up to 3 days, or freeze for up to 1 month. Divide the pickled vegetables among 3 small resealable bags, seal, label, and refrigerate for up to 5 days.

REHEAT FROM THE FRIDGE: Transfer the meatloaves to an oven-safe baking pan, add 2 tablespoons water, and tightly wrap the pan with aluminum foil. Bake the meatloaf in a 350°F oven for about 20 minutes, until warmed through. Or, place the meatloaf on a microwave-safe plate and cover with a damp paper towel. Microwave on low power for about 3 minutes, until warmed through. Serve with the pickled vegetables.

REHEAT FROM THE FREEZER: To thaw, place the meatloaf in the fridge overnight. Follow the instructions for reheating and serving from the fridge.

MIX IT UP: Want more flavor in your pickled veggies? Add 1 dill sprig and 1 teaspoon each of coriander seeds, celery seeds, and black peppercorns. Before serving, taste and season with salt, if needed.

Per Serving: Calories: 546; Total fat: 32g; Carbohydrates: 32g; Cholesterol: 100mg; Fiber: 2g; Protein: 30g; Sugar: 16g

Mediterranean Grilled Green Goddess Chicken Salad

Makes 3 servings

The garlicky, zesty flavors of the Mediterranean come together deliciously in this salad. Marinating the chicken in the dressing before grilling makes it super moist. For added crunch, I sometimes top the salad with chopped roasted almonds or cashews.

PREP TIME: 15 minutes, plus 15 minutes to marinate

COOK TIME: 8 minutes

1½ cups Green Goddess Dressing (page 105)
6 boneless, skinless chicken thighs (about 1 pound)
1 English cucumber, thinly sliced crosswise
3 tablespoons minced red onion
Fresh basil leaves, for serving
Salt (optional)
Freshly ground black pepper (optional)

1. Reserve 6 tablespoons of the dressing. Transfer the remaining dressing to a large resealable bag to serve as a marinade.

2. Place a large piece of plastic wrap or parchment paper on a work surface and put the chicken thighs on it. Cover with another piece of plastic wrap. Using a meat mallet or other heavy object, such as a rolling pin or cast-iron skillet, flatten each chicken thigh to about ½-inch thickness. Add the chicken to the bag with the marinade. Seal the bag and turn to coat the chicken well. Let sit at least 15 minutes, or refrigerate for up to 4 hours.

3. Preheat a grill or grill pan to medium heat.

62

4. Drain the chicken and place it on the grill. Reserve the marinade. Cook the chicken for 8 to 10 minutes, basting occasionally with the marinade. Then, flip the chicken and cook for another 5 minutes, basting a few more times with the marinade, until the chicken is cooked through and the juices run clear.

STORAGE: Cut the chicken into slices, then evenly divide it among 3 medium resealable containers. Cover, label, and refrigerate for up to 3 days. Divide the 6 tablespoons reserved dressing among 3 small resealable containers. Cover, label, and refrigerate for up to 5 days. Divide the cucumber and red onion among 3 small resealable bags, seal, label, and refrigerate for up to 3 days. Wrap the basil in damp paper towels and refrigerate for up to 3 days.

TO SERVE FROM THE FRIDGE: Place the chicken in a bowl. Add the cucumber and red onion, then pour on the dressing and toss to coat the chicken. Season with salt and pepper, if needed. Top with the basil leaves.

MIX IT UP: For a heartier meal, swap in beef for the chicken.

Per Serving: Calories: 476; Total fat: 30g; Carbohydrates: 11g; Cholesterol: 190mg; Fiber: 4g; Protein: 45g; Sugar: 2g

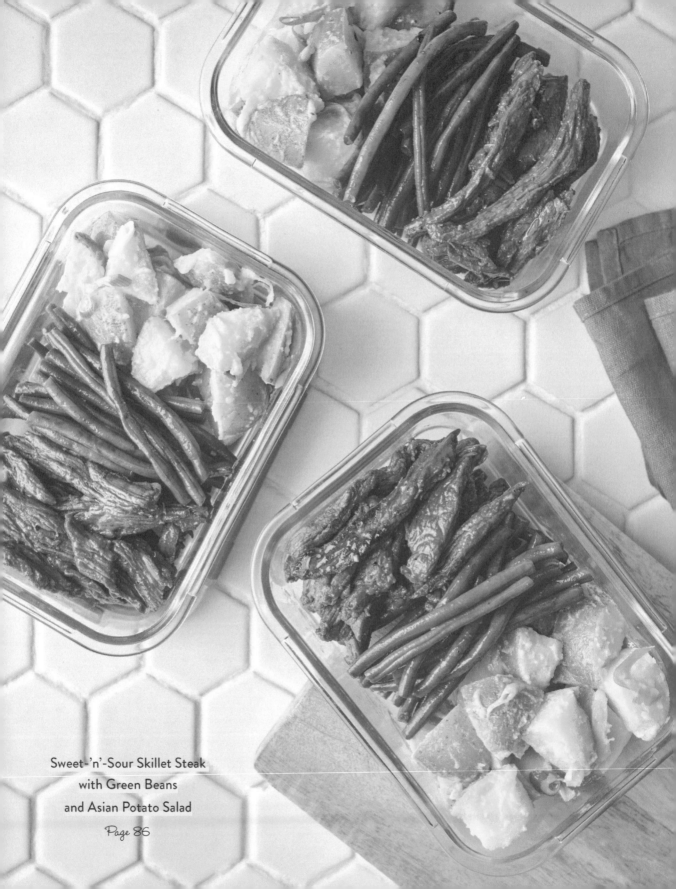

Sweet-'n'-Sour Skillet Steak
with Green Beans
and Asian Potato Salad

Page 86

Chapter Five

PREPPIN' PRO, WEEKS 5 AND 6

✳ ✳ ✳

Meal prep is in full swing—we're now prepping five meals each week. Oats are in the breakfast spotlight, both in cookie form with apples and cinnamon and as overnight oats with roasted fruit. Each week features both meat-filled—think Quick Pulled Pork Barbecue Sandwich with Tangy Cucumber Salad (page 74) and Sweet-'n'-Sour Skillet Steak with Green Beans and Asian Potato Salad (page 86)—and hearty vegan meals, like Zucchini Zoodles with Creamy Pesto Sauce (page 71) and Smoky Loaded Sweet Potato Soup (page 83). You'll also find fun, easy snacks, like Garlic Bread Popcorn (page 88) and Honey-Roasted Peanut and Pretzel Caramel Corn Crunch (page 76).

WEEK 5 RECIPES

Apple-Cinnamon Oatmeal Breakfast Cookies

Zucchini Zoodles with Creamy Pesto Sauce

Scallion-Ginger Noodles with Pork

Quick Pulled Pork Barbecue Sandwich with Tangy Cucumber Salad

Honey-Roasted Peanut and Pretzel Caramel Corn Crunch

WEEK 5 SHOPPING LIST

CANNED AND BOTTLED ITEMS
- ☐ Applesauce, unsweetened chunky, 1 (24-ounce) jar
- ☐ Barbecue sauce, 1 (8-ounce) jar
- ☐ Broth, chicken, 1 (14-ounce) can

DAIRY ALTERNATIVES AND EGGS
- ☐ Butter, Dairy-Free (page 96), or store-bought dairy-free (½ cup)
- ☐ Cheese, Grated Parmesan (page 99), or store-bought dairy-free parmesan-style (6 tablespoons)
- ☐ Egg, large (1)
- ☐ Milk, Cashew (page 94), or store-bought dairy-free (2 tablespoons)

MEAT
- ☐ Pork tenderloin, boneless (1½ pounds)

PANTRY INGREDIENTS
- ☐ Apples, chopped dried (½ cup)
- ☐ Baking powder
- ☐ Baking soda
- ☐ Chili powder
- ☐ Cinnamon, ground
- ☐ Flour, all-purpose or gluten-free
- ☐ Honey (¾ cup)
- ☐ Oats, quick-cooking or certified gluten-free (1½ cups)
- ☐ Oil, olive (10 tablespoons)
- ☐ Oil, vegetable (10 tablespoons)
- ☐ Peanuts, unsalted roasted (1 cup)
- ☐ Pepper, freshly ground black
- ☐ Popcorn, unsalted popped (5 cups)
- ☐ Pretzels, mini or gluten-free (1 cup)
- ☐ Salt
- ☐ Spaghetti, regular or gluten-free (6 ounces)
- ☐ Sugar, granulated
- ☐ Sugar, light brown (¼ cup)

- ☐ Syrup, brown rice (2 tablespoons) or corn syrup
- ☐ Tamari
- ☐ Vanilla extract
- ☐ Vinegar, apple cider (6 tablespoons)
- ☐ Walnuts (1 cup)

PRODUCE
- ☐ Basil (2 or 3 bunches)
- ☐ Bell pepper, red (1)
- ☐ Broccoli, head (1½ pounds; 3 cups trimmed florets)
- ☐ Dill (1 bunch)
- ☐ English cucumbers (2)
- ☐ Garlic (1 head)
- ☐ Ginger (1-inch piece)
- ☐ Lemon (1)
- ☐ Lettuce, romaine (1)
- ☐ Onions, red (2)
- ☐ Scallions (1 bunch)
- ☐ Zucchini (3 pounds)

OTHER
- ☐ Sandwich buns, regular or gluten-free potato (3)

SPECIAL EQUIPMENT
- ☐ Candy thermometer (optional)
- ☐ Food processor or blender
- ☐ Ice cream scoop, small (optional)
- ☐ Mixer, handheld electric (optional)
- ☐ Spiralizer or vegetable peeler

WEEK 5 STEP-BY-STEP PREP

1. Preheat the oven to 350°F. Make the Apple-Cinnamon Oatmeal Breakfast Cookies (page 70). Package 4 cookies each in 5 small resealable containers, cover, and store at room temperature.

2. Cook the pork for the Quick Pulled Pork Barbecue Sandwich with Tangy Cucumber Salad (page 74). Shred the pork and combine with the barbecue sauce. Evenly divide the pork among 3 small resealable microwave-safe containers. Cover, label, and refrigerate.

3. Make the cucumber salad for the Quick Pulled Pork Barbecue Sandwich with Tangy Cucumber Salad (page 74). Evenly divide the cucumber salad among 3 small resealable containers. Cover, label, and refrigerate. Place 1 bun in each of 3 resealable bags, seal, and store at room temperature.

4. Make the Zucchini Zoodles with Creamy Pesto Sauce (page 71). Divide the zoodles among 4 medium resealable microwave-safe containers. Top each with ½ cup sauce and place in the fridge.

Continues →

5. Prepare the Scallion-Ginger
Noodles with Pork (page 72).
Evenly divide the pork and noodles among 3 medium resealable
microwave-safe containers. Cover,
label, and refrigerate. Evenly
divide the scallion greens among
3 small resealable bags; seal, label,
and refrigerate.

6. Make the Honey-Roasted Peanut
and Pretzel Caramel Corn Crunch
(page 76). Evenly divide among
5 medium resealable containers, cover, and store at room
temperature.

WEEK 5 MEAL PLAN

	BREAKFAST	LUNCH	DINNER	SNACK
DAY 1	Apple-Cinnamon Oatmeal Breakfast Cookies	Quick Pulled Pork Barbecue Sandwich with Tangy Cucumber Salad	Zucchini Zoodles with Creamy Pesto Sauce	Honey-Roasted Peanut and Pretzel Caramel Corn Crunch
DAY 2	Apple-Cinnamon Oatmeal Breakfast Cookies	Scallion-Ginger Noodles with Pork	Quick Pulled Pork Barbecue Sandwich with Tangy Cucumber Salad	Honey-Roasted Peanut and Pretzel Caramel Corn Crunch
DAY 3	Apple-Cinnamon Oatmeal Breakfast Cookies	Zucchini Zoodles with Creamy Pesto Sauce	Scallion-Ginger Noodles with Pork	Honey-Roasted Peanut and Pretzel Caramel Corn Crunch
DAY 4	Apple-Cinnamon Oatmeal Breakfast Cookies	Quick Pulled Pork Barbecue Sandwich with Tangy Cucumber Salad	Zucchini Zoodles with Creamy Pesto Sauce	Honey-Roasted Peanut and Pretzel Caramel Corn Crunch
DAY 5	Apple-Cinnamon Oatmeal Breakfast Cookies	Zucchini Zoodles with Creamy Pesto Sauce	Scallion-Ginger Noodles with Pork	Honey-Roasted Peanut and Pretzel Caramel Corn Crunch

Apple-Cinnamon Oatmeal Breakfast Cookies

Makes about 20 cookies

This is a breakfast cookie you can feel good about, with its protein-packed oats and a double dose of fiber-rich apples— as dried apples and as applesauce.

PREP TIME: 15 minutes

COOK TIME: 18 minutes

1½ cups quick-cooking rolled oats or certified gluten-free old-fashioned rolled oats

1 cup all-purpose flour or gluten-free flour

½ cup chopped dried apples

1 teaspoon baking powder

¾ teaspoon ground cinnamon

½ teaspoon salt

¼ teaspoon baking soda

½ cup Dairy-Free Butter (page 96) or store-bought dairy-free butter, at room temperature

¼ cup granulated sugar

¼ cup packed light brown sugar

1 large egg, at room temperature

¾ cup unsweetened chunky applesauce

1 teaspoon vanilla extract

1. Preheat the oven to 350°F. Line 2 baking sheets with parchment paper.

2. In a medium bowl, whisk the oats, flour, dried apples, baking powder, cinnamon, salt, and baking soda to combine.

3. In a large bowl, use a handheld electric mixer (or whisk) to cream the butter and sugars on medium-high speed until smooth.

4. Add the egg to the butter-sugar mixture and mix on medium speed until combined. Stir in the applesauce, vanilla, and the flour mixture until combined. Using a small ice cream scoop or tablespoon measure, drop the batter (by 1½ tablespoons) onto the prepared baking sheets and flatten slightly.

5. Bake for about 18 minutes, until golden around the edges. Transfer to a wire rack and let cool completely.

> **STORAGE:** Package 4 cookies each in 5 small resealable containers, cover, and store at room temperature for up to 5 days.
>
> **MIX IT UP:** If you want some nuttiness, stir ½ cup chopped walnuts in step 4.

Per Serving (4 cookies): Calories: 456; Total fat: 21g; Carbohydrates: 61g; Cholesterol: 37mg; Fiber: 6g; Protein: 7g; Sugar: 25g

Zucchini Zoodles with Creamy Pesto Sauce

Makes 4 servings

For cheesiness here, I use homemade Grated Parmesan Cheese (page 99), but you can also use nutritional yeast if you have some on hand.

PREP TIME: 20 minutes

FOR THE PESTO SAUCE

2 cups fresh basil leaves

2 garlic cloves, peeled

1 cup walnuts

½ cup olive oil

6 tablespoons Grated Parmesan Cheese (page 99) or store-bought dairy-free parmesan-style grated cheese

2 tablespoons freshly squeezed lemon juice (from 1 lemon)

½ teaspoon salt

1 tablespoon water, plus more as needed

FOR THE ZUCCHINI ZOODLES

3 pounds zucchini, stem ends trimmed

½ teaspoon salt

TO MAKE THE PESTO SAUCE

1. In a food processor or blender, combine the basil, garlic, walnuts, olive oil, parmesan, lemon juice, and salt. Process until smooth. Add the water, 1 tablespoon at a time, and process until creamy.

TO MAKE THE ZUCCHINI ZOODLES

2. Using a spiralizer or vegetable peeler, create strips of zucchini as thin as possible.

3. Place the zucchini zoodles in a colander. Sprinkle on the salt and toss to combine. Place the colander in a clean sink or over a bowl and let drain for 5 minutes, until the zucchini has released its liquid. Pat dry.

STORAGE: Divide the zoodles among 4 medium resealable microwave-safe containers. Top each with ½ cup pesto sauce. Cover, label, and refrigerate for up to 4 days.

REHEAT FROM THE FRIDGE: Remove the lid on the container and microwave on high power for 2 to 3 minutes, until warmed through.

MIX IT UP: Swap in thin strips of carrot or beet zoodles for the zucchini.

Scallion-Ginger Noodles with Pork

Makes 3 servings

The noodles here are a vehicle for this gingery, oniony, simple
weeknight ramen-style dish that's sweetened with a bit of honey.
In place of the classic Asian ramen noodles, I use spaghetti
for convenience, as it is always in my pantry.

PREP TIME: 15 minutes

COOK TIME: 15 minutes

Salt

6 ounces regular or gluten-free spaghetti

10 tablespoons vegetable oil, divided, plus
more for coating

1 small pork tenderloin (about 12 ounces),
cut into ½-inch cubes

Freshly ground black pepper

3 cups fresh broccoli florets (about
1¼ pounds)

1 red bell pepper, seeded and thinly sliced

2 garlic cloves

1 (1-inch) piece fresh ginger, peeled and
finely chopped

2 scallions, trimmed, green and white parts
finely chopped

2 to 4 tablespoons water

3 tablespoons apple cider vinegar

1½ tablespoons honey

1 tablespoon tamari

1 head romaine lettuce, trimmed and cut
crosswise

1. Bring a medium pot of salted
   water to a boil over high heat. Add
   the spaghetti and cook for about
   8 minutes, until al dente. Drain in
   a colander and toss in a bowl with
   a little vegetable oil to lightly coat.

2. In a large skillet over medium-high
   heat, heat 2 tablespoons of the
   vegetable oil until shimmering,
   about 1 minute. Add the pork and
   sauté for about 5 minutes, until
   lightly browned. Season with salt
   and pepper, then transfer to a
   medium bowl.

3. Add 2 more tablespoons of vegetable oil to the skillet, followed
   by the broccoli, bell pepper, garlic,
   ginger, and scallions. Cook for
   about 2 minutes, stirring occasionally, until the vegetables start
   to soften, adding a little water,
   1 tablespoon at a time, if necessary.
   Season with salt and pepper.

72

4. In a large bowl, whisk the vinegar, honey, tamari, and remaining
    6 tablespoons vegetable oil until emulsified. Add the spaghetti, vegetable
    mixture from the skillet, and the romaine strips. Toss to coat well, and season
    to taste with salt and pepper.

STORAGE: Evenly divide the pork and noodles among 3 medium resealable microwave-safe containers. Cover, label, and refrigerate for up to 4 days.

REHEAT FROM THE FRIDGE: Remove the lid from the container and microwave on high power for about 3 minutes, until warmed through.

INGREDIENT TIP: Omit the pork to make this dish vegetarian.

Per Serving: Calories 862; Total fat 52g; Carbohydrates 71g; Cholesterol 65mg; Fiber 8g; Protein 34g; Sugar 17g

Quick Pulled Pork Barbecue Sandwich with Tangy Cucumber Salad

Makes 3 servings

The secret to making barbecue pulled pork easily and quickly is to start with pork tenderloin, a quick-cooking cut that takes just 20 minutes to get tender enough to be shredded and stirred with barbecue sauce. The cucumber salad here gets its nice tang from a quick pickling.

PREP TIME: 20 minutes

COOK TIME: 30 minutes

FOR THE CUCUMBER SALAD

3 tablespoons apple cider vinegar

1½ tablespoons olive oil

½ tablespoon chopped fresh dill

Sugar (optional)

Salt

Freshly ground black pepper

1½ English cucumbers, thinly sliced

½ red onion, sliced

FOR THE PORK

12 ounces pork tenderloin, cut crosswise into 1½-inch-thick slices

Olive oil

Salt

Freshly ground black pepper

Regular or gluten-free Chili powder, for seasoning

1½ cups regular or gluten-free chicken broth

¾ cup barbecue sauce of choice

3 sandwich buns or gluten-free potato buns, split in half, for serving

TO MAKE THE CUCUMBER SALAD

1. In a large bowl, whisk together the vinegar, olive oil, and dill. Season with a pinch of sugar (if using), salt, and pepper. Whisk again, then stir in the cucumbers and red onion. Toss to coat everything well with the dressing.

TO MAKE THE PORK

2. Rub the pork generously with some olive oil and season all over with salt, pepper, and chili powder.

3. In a small Dutch oven set over medium-high heat, bring the chicken broth to a boil. Add the pork and reduce the heat to a simmer. Cover the pot and cook for 15 to 20 minutes, until the meat is just cooked through. Transfer the pork slices to a cutting board and let rest for 3 minutes.

74

4. Using two forks, shred the pork into bite-size pieces. Return the meat to the pot and adjust the heat to medium.

5. Stir in the barbecue sauce, and cook for about 3 minutes, until the meat is heated through. Season to taste with salt and pepper.

STORAGE: Let the pork cool slightly. Evenly divide the pork among 3 small resealable microwave-safe containers. Cover, label, and refrigerate for up to 4 days. Evenly divide the cucumber salad among 3 small resealable containers. Cover, label, and refrigerate for up to 4 days. Place 1 bun in each of 3 resealable bags, seal, label, and refrigerate for up to 4 days.

REHEAT FROM THE FRIDGE: Remove the lid from the pork container and microwave on high power for about 2 minutes, until warmed through, adding a little water, 1 tablespoon at a time, if needed, to thin the sauce a bit. Spoon the pork onto the bun bottom and place the bun top alongside. Serve the cucumber salad either on the sandwich or on the side.

MIX IT UP: Want some heat? Add some thinly sliced jalapeño to the cucumber salad.

Per Serving: Calories: 491 Total fat: 19g Carbohydrates: 53g Cholesterol: 65mg Fiber: 3g Protein: 28g Sugar: 23g

Honey-Roasted Peanut and Pretzel Caramel Corn Crunch

Makes 5 servings

You'll never buy store-bought caramel corn again. This recipe is super easy and ready in minutes—not to mention slightly addictive, with its salty-sweet combination of honey, pretzels, popcorn, and peanuts.

PREP TIME: 12 minutes

COOK TIME: 10 minutes

5 cups unsalted popped popcorn
1 cup regular or gluten-free mini pretzels
1 cup sugar
¼ cup honey
2 tablespoons brown rice syrup or corn syrup
1 cup unsalted roasted peanuts
Salt

1. Line a baking sheet with parchment paper. Set aside.

2. In a large heatproof bowl, combine the popcorn and pretzels.

3. In a small saucepan over medium-high heat, combine the sugar, honey, syrup, and peanuts. Cook for about 10 minutes, stirring occasionally, until a candy thermometer registers 290°F (soft-crack stage; see tip). Working quickly, pour the sugar mixture over the popcorn and pretzels, and stir to coat everything with the caramel. Transfer the mixture to the prepared baking sheet, spreading it out to an even thickness. Sprinkle to taste with salt. Let cool completely.

STORAGE: Evenly divide the mix among 5 medium resealable containers, cover, and store at room temperature for up to 5 days.

COOKING TIP: If you don't own a candy thermometer, or even if you do, you'll know the sugar mixture is ready when the color turns golden brown.

Per Serving: Calories: 519; Total fat: 15g; Carbohydrates: 93g; Cholesterol: 0mg; Fiber: 6g; Protein: 11g; Sugar: 57g

WEEK 6 RECIPES

Overnight Oats Breakfast Bowl with Roasted Fruit

Smoky Loaded Sweet Potato Soup

Pasta with Rosemary, Bean, and Bacon Ragout

Sweet-'n'-Sour Skillet Steak with Green Beans and Asian Potato Salad

Garlic Bread Popcorn

WEEK 6 SHOPPING LIST

CANNED AND BOTTLED ITEMS
- ☐ Beans, cannellini, 1 (15-ounce) can
- ☐ Broth, chicken, 1 (14-ounce) can
- ☐ Chipotle chiles in adobo sauce, 1 (7-ounce) can

DAIRY ALTERNATIVES AND EGGS
- ☐ Butter, Dairy-Free (page 96), or store-bought dairy-free (2 tablespoons)
- ☐ Cheese, Grated Parmesan (page 99), or store-bought dairy-free parmesan-style (2 tablespoons)
- ☐ Milk, Cashew (page 94), or store-bought dairy-free (2 tablespoons)

MEAT
- ☐ Bacon (8 ounces)
- ☐ Steak, skirt (12 ounces)

PANTRY INGREDIENTS
- ☐ Cinnamon, ground
- ☐ Ketchup
- ☐ Macaroni, regular or gluten-free (12 ounces)
- ☐ Mustard, Dijon
- ☐ Oats, old-fashioned rolled or certified gluten-free (1½ cups)
- ☐ Oil, olive (1 cup)
- ☐ Pecans, chopped (¼ cup)
- ☐ Pepper, freshly ground black
- ☐ Popcorn, unsalted popped (6 cups)
- ☐ Pumpkin seeds (¼ cup)
- ☐ Raisins (¼ cup)
- ☐ Salt
- ☐ Sugar
- ☐ Tamari
- ☐ Vinegar, apple cider

PRODUCE

- ☐ Apples (3)
- ☐ Carrot (1)
- ☐ Chives (1 small bunch)
- ☐ Escarole (1 head)
- ☐ Garlic (1 small head)
- ☐ Green beans (12 ounces)
- ☐ Lemon (1)
- ☐ Onion (1 small)
- ☐ Orange (1)
- ☐ Parsley, flat-leaf (1 small bunch)
- ☐ Pears (3)
- ☐ Potatoes, new red (1½ pounds)
- ☐ Rosemary (1 small bunch)
- ☐ Scallions (1 bunch)
- ☐ Sweet potatoes (2)

SPECIAL EQUIPMENT

- ☐ Blender, high-speed

WEEK 6 STEP-BY-STEP PREP

1. If using, make the Cashew Milk (page 94) and then the Dairy-Free Butter (page 96) for the Overnight Oats Breakfast Bowl with Roasted Fruit (page 81). Refrigerate both items in airtight containers.

2. Preheat the oven to 425°F. Make the roasted fruit for the Overnight Oats Breakfast Bowl with Roasted Fruit (page 81).

3. Make the Smoky Loaded Sweet Potato Soup (page 83). Divide among 3 medium resealable microwave-safe containers. Cover, label, and refrigerate.

4. Make the overnight oats for the Overnight Oats Breakfast Bowl with Roasted Fruit (page 81). Divide the oats among 5 small resealable containers. Top each with one-fifth of the cooled fruit, cover, label, and place in the fridge.

5. Make the Pasta with Rosemary, Bean, and Bacon Ragout (page 84). Divide the ragout among 4 medium resealable microwave-safe containers. Cover, label, and refrigerate.

6. Make the Sweet-'n'-Sour Skillet Steak with Green Beans and Asian Potato Salad (page 86). Divide the potato salad among 3 medium resealable microwave-safe containers and top with the steak and green beans. Cover, label, and store in the fridge.

7. If using, make the Grated Parmesan Cheese (page 99) for the Garlic Bread Popcorn (page 88). Refrigerate in an airtight container.

8. Make the Garlic Bread Popcorn (page 88). Divide the popcorn among 5 medium resealable bags, seal, and store at room temperature.

WEEK 6 MEAL PLAN

	BREAKFAST	LUNCH	DINNER	SNACK
DAY 1	Overnight Oats Breakfast Bowl with Roasted Fruit	Pasta with Rosemary, Bean, and Bacon Ragout	Sweet-'n'-Sour Skillet Steak with Green Beans and Asian Potato Salad	Garlic Bread Popcorn
DAY 2	Overnight Oats Breakfast Bowl with Roasted Fruit	Smoky Loaded Sweet Potato Soup	Pasta with Rosemary, Bean, and Bacon Ragout	Garlic Bread Popcorn
DAY 3	Overnight Oats Breakfast Bowl with Roasted Fruit	Sweet-'n'-Sour Skillet Steak with Green Beans and Asian Potato Salad	Smoky Loaded Sweet Potato Soup	Garlic Bread Popcorn
DAY 4	Overnight Oats Breakfast Bowl with Roasted Fruit	Pasta with Rosemary, Bean, and Bacon Ragout	Sweet-'n'-Sour Skillet Steak with Green Beans and Asian Potato Salad	Garlic Bread Popcorn
DAY 5	Overnight Oats Breakfast Bowl with Roasted Fruit	Smoky Loaded Sweet Potato Soup	Pasta with Rosemary, Bean, and Bacon Ragout	Garlic Bread Popcorn

Overnight Oats Breakfast Bowl with Roasted Fruit

Makes 5 servings

I've been making overnight oats for years, because they give me a burst of energy to start my day. Roasting the fruit intensifies its flavor, a step that takes this otherwise humble breakfast to a whole new level.

PREP TIME: 15 minutes plus overnight

COOK TIME: 20 minutes

FOR THE ROASTED FRUIT

¼ cup raisins

Hot water

3 apples, halved, cored, and cut into small chunks

3 pears, halved, cored, and cut into small chunks

Grated zest of 1 lemon

Juice of 1 lemon

¼ cup chopped pecans

¼ cup pumpkin seeds

¼ cup sugar

½ teaspoon ground cinnamon

2 tablespoons Dairy-Free Butter (page 96) or store-bought dairy-free butter

FOR THE OVERNIGHT OATS

1½ cups old-fashioned rolled oats or certified gluten-free oats

1¼ cups water

Grated zest of 1 orange

Juice of 1 orange (about ¼ cup)

¼ teaspoon salt

TO MAKE THE ROASTED FRUIT

1. Preheat the oven to 425°F.

2. In a small bowl, combine the raisins with enough hot water to cover. Let soak for at least 15 minutes. Drain.

3. On a baking sheet, combine the apples, pears, lemon zest, lemon juice, pecans, and pumpkin seeds. Toss to combine.

4. Sprinkle the sugar and cinnamon on top. Dot with the butter.

5. Roast for 15 to 20 minutes, turning once, until golden.

6. Pour into a bowl and stir in the raisins. Let the roasted fruit cool completely.

TO MAKE THE OVERNIGHT OATS

7. In a large bowl, stir together the oats, water, orange zest, orange juice, and salt. Cover the bowl and refrigerate overnight.

81

Continues →

STORAGE: Divide the oats among 5 small resealable containers. Top each with one-fifth of the fruit mixture. Cover, label, and refrigerate for up to 5 days.

SUBSTITUTION TIP: Swap in your favorite nuts and seeds for the pecans and pumpkin seeds, or swap in your favorite berries for the apples and pears.

Per Serving: Calories: 413; Total fat: 13g; Carbohydrates: 73g; Cholesterol: 0mg; Fiber: 11g; Protein: 7g; Sugar: 42g

82

Smoky Loaded Sweet Potato Soup

Makes 3 servings

This 15-minute blender soup gets its smokiness from the bacon and the chipotle chiles in adobo sauce. The fiber-rich sweet potatoes lend a wonderful, starchy creaminess, while the carrots offer a hint of sweetness. If you want to make this soup vegan, just omit the bacon.

PREP TIME: 15 minutes

COOK TIME: 20 minutes

2 sweet potatoes (about 1 pound), peeled and chopped

2 bacon slices, chopped

1 small onion, chopped

1 carrot, shredded

1 canned chipotle chile in adobo sauce, plus 1½ teaspoons adobo sauce

1 cup water

Salt

Freshly ground black pepper

2 tablespoons finely chopped fresh chives

STORAGE: Evenly divide the soup among 3 resealable microwave-safe containers. Cover, label, and refrigerate for up to 5 days. Evenly divide the chives among 3 small resealable bags, seal, label, and refrigerate for up to 5 days.

REHEAT FROM THE FRIDGE: Remove the lid on the container of soup and microwave on high power for about 3 minutes, until warmed through. Serve with the chives.

1. In a medium pot, combine the sweet potatoes and enough water just to cover. Place the pot over high heat and bring to a boil. Cook for about 15 minutes, until the sweet potatoes are tender when pierced with a fork. Drain.

2. In a small skillet over medium-high heat, cook the bacon for about 5 minutes, until the fat renders. Add the onion and carrot. Cook for about 10 minutes, stirring occasionally, until the vegetables have softened. Transfer the bacon, onion, and carrot to a high-speed blender.

3. Add the sweet potato, chipotle chile, adobo sauce, and the water to the blender. Blend on high speed until smooth, about 1 minute. Taste and adjust the seasoning with salt and pepper. Let the soup cool slightly.

83

Per Serving: Calories 227 Total Fat 6g Carbohydrates 38g Cholesterol 14mg Fiber 6g Protein 6g Sugar 10g

Pasta with Rosemary, Bean, and Bacon Ragout

Makes 4 servings

I spent dozens of my childhood summers with my Italian grandfather, cooking with him in his Roman kitchen. This hearty dish is a take on his traditional Italian pasta e fagioli, or pasta with beans.

PREP TIME: 10 minutes

COOK TIME: 20 minutes

Salt

12 ounces (about 3 cups) regular or gluten-free macaroni

2 bacon slices, chopped

1 head escarole, cored, halved, and cut into strips

1 tablespoon chopped fresh rosemary

2 garlic cloves, smashed

½ cup regular or gluten-free chicken broth or water

1 (15-ounce) can regular or gluten-free cannellini beans, rinsed and drained

1. Bring a large pot of salted water to a boil over high heat. Add the macaroni and cook for about 9 minutes, until al dente. Reserve ¼ cup of the pasta cooking water, then drain the pasta.

2. In a medium saucepan over medium-high heat, cook the bacon for about 6 minutes, until the fat renders. Add the escarole, rosemary, and garlic. Cook for about 4 minutes, until the escarole is wilted and the garlic is softened.

3. Add the broth and beans. Cook for about 5 minutes, until the beans are warmed through. Taste and season with salt.

4. Place the macaroni in a large bowl and add the bean ragout. Stir well and add enough of the reserved pasta cooking water to provide a little broth. Let cool.

STORAGE: Divide the ragout among 4 medium resealable microwave-safe containers. Cover, label, and refrigerate for up to 4 days.

REHEAT FROM THE FRIDGE: Remove the lid on the ragout container and microwave on high power for about 3 minutes, until warmed through.

INGREDIENT TIP: Feeling fancy? Top the ragout with about 1 pound cooked medium shrimp.

Per Serving: Calories: 463; Total fat: 6g; Carbohydrates: 80g; Cholesterol: 10mg; Fiber: 9g; Protein: 20g; Sugar: 6g

Sweet-'n'-Sour Skillet Steak with Green Beans and Asian Potato Salad

Makes 3 servings

I have put an Asian-inspired twist on the classic American steak and potatoes. In place of the mashed or baked potatoes, I have a mayonnaise-free potato salad with a mustardy, scallion dressing. The steak is seasoned with a sweet-and-sour garlicky tamari marinade that features a classic American "secret" ingredient—ketchup.

PREP TIME: 20 minutes

COOK TIME: 30 minutes

FOR THE POTATO SALAD

1½ pounds red new potatoes, cut into
   1-inch pieces

Salt

1½ tablespoons apple cider vinegar

1½ teaspoons Dijon mustard

½ teaspoon sugar

1½ scallions, trimmed, white and green
   parts finely chopped

3 tablespoons olive oil, plus more for
   drizzling

Freshly ground black pepper

FOR THE STEAK AND GREEN BEANS

2 tablespoons ketchup

1½ tablespoons tamari

1 tablespoon apple cider vinegar

2 teaspoons sugar

1 garlic clove, finely chopped

12 ounces skirt steak, cut into 4-inch-wide
   pieces, then cut against the grain into
   ¼-inch-thick slices

Salt

Freshly ground black pepper

2 teaspoons olive oil, plus more as needed

12 ounces fresh green beans, ends trimmed

1½ tablespoons water

TO MAKE THE POTATO SALAD

1. Place the potatoes in a large pot of salted water. Put the pot over medium heat and bring to a boil, then reduce the heat to low and simmer for about 10 minutes or until the potatoes are fork-tender. Drain and transfer the potatoes to a medium bowl.

2. Whisk the vinegar, mustard, sugar, and scallions in a small bowl. Add the olive oil in a slow, steady stream until blended and emulsified.

3. Pour the dressing over the potatoes and gently toss to coat with the dressing. Season to taste with salt and pepper.

TO MAKE THE STEAK AND GREEN BEANS

4. In a medium bowl, whisk together the ketchup, tamari, vinegar, sugar, and garlic.

5. Season the steak all over with salt and pepper. Add the meat to the ketchup mixture and toss to coat well.

6. In a large skillet over medium-high heat, heat the olive oil. Add the meat and sauté for about 4 minutes or until it's cooked through. Transfer to a plate.

7. Return the skillet to the heat and add the beans, adding more oil if needed. Sprinkle in the water and cover the skillet. Steam over medium heat for 5 minutes, then uncover the skillet and cook for about 5 minutes more, until the beans are crisp-tender.

8. Return the beef and any accumulated juices to the skillet with the beans. Toss to combine and then let cool.

STORAGE: Divide the potato salad among 3 medium resealable microwave-safe containers and top with the steak and green beans. Cover, label, and refrigerate for up to 5 days.

REHEAT FROM THE FRIDGE: Remove the lid from the container and microwave on high power for about 3 minutes, until warmed through.

SUBSTITUTION TIP: For a more authentic flavor, use Kewpie mayo (available on Amazon), which has a wonderful umami taste.

Per Serving: Calories: 568; Total fat: 28g; Carbohydrates: 51g; Cholesterol: 90mg; Fiber: 10g; Protein: 32g; Sugar: 10g

Garlic Bread Popcorn

Makes 5 servings

This recipe brings the classic flavors of garlic bread—garlic, parmesan cheese, and parsley—to popcorn. This easy-to-make savory snack is great for an afternoon pick-me-up or for binge-watching your favorite new show.

PREP TIME: 5 minutes

COOK TIME: 2 minutes

6 cups unsalted popped popcorn

3 tablespoons olive oil

1½ teaspoons finely chopped garlic

1 tablespoon finely chopped fresh flat-leaf parsley

⅛ teaspoon salt

1 tablespoon Grated Parmesan Cheese (page 99) or store-bought dairy-free parmesan-style cheese

1. Place the popcorn in a large bowl.

2. In a small saucepan over medium heat, heat the olive oil. Add the garlic, parsley, and salt. Cook for about 2 minutes, stirring occasionally, until warmed, then drizzle the seasoned oil over the popcorn.

3. Sprinkle the popcorn with the cheese and toss to coat well. Let cool completely.

STORAGE: Divide the popcorn among 5 medium resealable bags. Seal and store at room temperature for up to 5 days.

SUBSTITUTION TIP: Do you like popping your own popcorn? If so, substitute ¼ cup popcorn kernels and pop them according to their package directions.

Per Serving: Calories: 189; Total fat: 10g; Carbohydrates: 23g; Cholesterol: 1mg; Fiber: 4g; Protein: 4g; Sugar: 0g

88

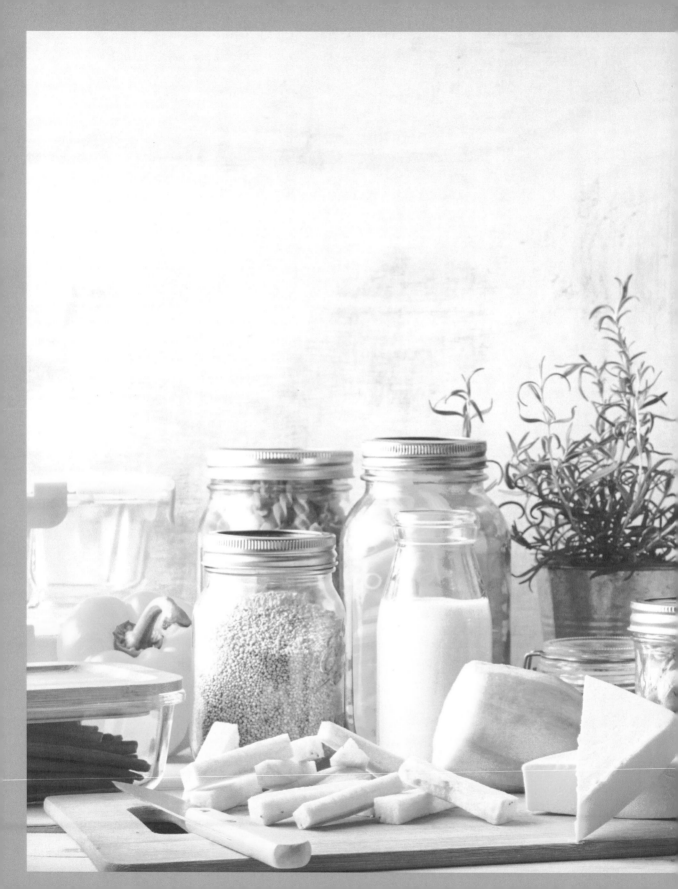

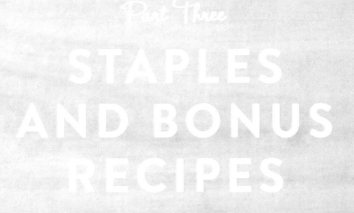

Part Three

STAPLES
AND BONUS
RECIPES

✳ ✳ ✳

Now that you're a meal-prep pro, you're ready to build a repertoire of basic dairy-free staples like milk, butter, parmesan, and cream cheese, as well as versatile creamy sauces and dressings. In this section, you'll be inspired by dozens of meal prep–friendly recipes for breakfast, lunch, dinner, sides, and snacks to mix up your weekly menus for the month. Mix and match your favorite recipes from all the preps to keep meals fun and interesting.

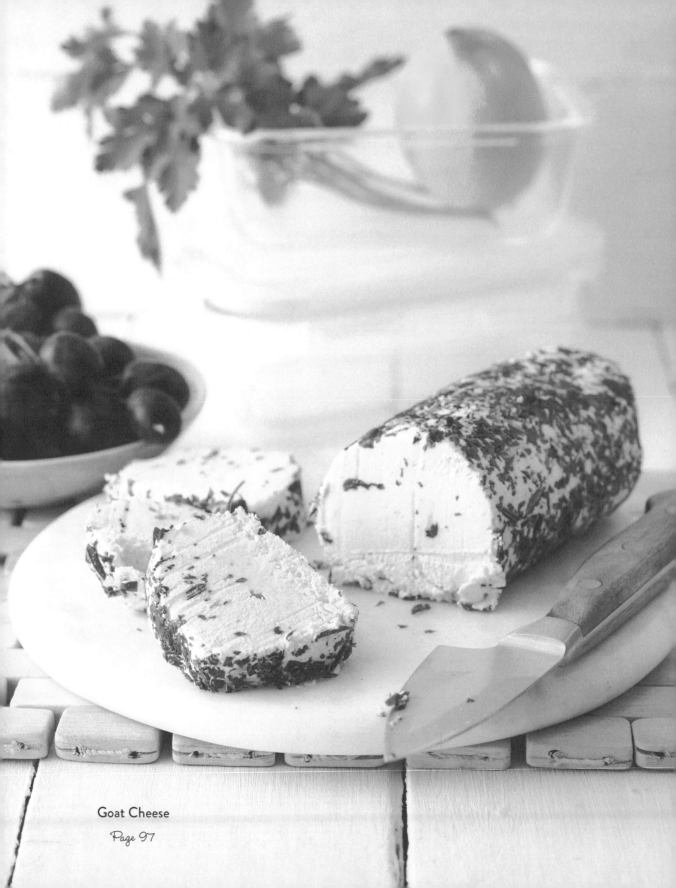

Goat Cheese

Page 97

Chapter Six

STAPLES AND SAUCES

※ ※ ※

Cashew Milk

Makes 4 cups

Of all the dairy-free milks on the market these days, including hemp, quinoa, hazelnut, almond, and coconut, cashew is my favorite— and homemade is even better than the supermarket version. In the kitchen, cashew milk is the most versatile nut milk because of its healthy high-fat content, which makes it ultra-creamy in texture without all the additives. A touch of date syrup replaces the lactose sugar found in cow's milk for a little sweetness, or use whatever sweetener you have in your pantry, including maple syrup, agave syrup, or even honey. If you prefer your milk unsweetened, leave out the syrup. This recipe makes low-fat milk. To make this recipe into heavy cream and/or buttermilk, see the ingredient tip that follows.

PREP TIME: 5 minutes, plus 4 hours to soak

1 cup raw cashews, soaked in water for at least 4 hours or overnight, then rinsed and drained

1 to 2 tablespoons date syrup (optional)

¼ teaspoon salt

4 cups water

In a high-speed blender, combine the cashews, date syrup (if using), salt, and water. Blend on high speed for about 1 minute, until smooth. Strain through a fine-mesh sieve into a medium bowl.

STORAGE: Refrigerate the milk in a 1-quart resealable container for up to 1 week.

VARIATION TIP: To make nonfat milk, use 5 cups water; to make whole-fat milk, use 3 cups water. To make heavy cream, use 2 to 2½ cups water plus 1 tablespoon avocado oil. To make buttermilk, stir 1 tablespoon apple cider vinegar into 1 cup of the cashew milk and keep refrigerated for up to 3 days.

Per Serving (1 cup): Calories: 25; Total fat: 2g; Carbohydrates: 1g; Cholesterol: 0mg; Fiber: 0g; Protein: 0g; Sugar: 0g

Oat Milk

Makes 4 cups

Oat milk is deliciously neutral in flavor and has a wonderful viscosity, which is accomplished by blending the milk with your favorite neutral-flavored oil. Adding the oil also makes the oat milk froth well for your morning cappuccino. For the sweetener, I love date syrup, but you can use whatever sweetener you have on hand.

PREP TIME: 5 minutes, plus 15 minutes to soak

1 cup steel-cut oats, soaked for 15 minutes, then rinsed and drained

1 to 2 tablespoons date syrup (optional; see tip)

Seeds from 1 vanilla bean, or 2 teaspoons vanilla extract (optional; see tip)

1 tablespoon neutral-flavored oil

¼ teaspoon salt

3 to 4 cups water

In a high-speed blender, combine the oats, date syrup (if using), vanilla (if using), oil, salt, and 3 cups water. Process on high speed until smooth, about 1 minute. Add some or all of the remaining 1 cup water to achieve your desired consistency. Strain through a coarse-mesh sieve into a medium bowl.

95

STORAGE: Store in a resealable container in the refrigerator for up to 1 week.

SUBSTITUTION TIP: If you're using the oat milk for cooking savory foods, leave out the syrup and vanilla.

Per Serving (1 cup) Calories 120 Total fat 5g Carbohydrates 16g Cholesterol 0mg Fiber 2g Protein 3g Sugar 4g

Dairy-Free Butter

Makes about 1 cup

It took me months to crack the code for a dairy-free butter that could spread, melt, and taste like the real deal. For this recipe, I use cacao butter, which is the cold-pressed oil of the cacao bean—and it's a healthy source of antioxidants and omega-6 and omega-9 fatty acids, as well. You can find cacao butter and sunflower lecithin at your local health food store or online.

PREP TIME: 5 minutes

¼ cup refined coconut oil, melted

2 tablespoons Cashew Milk (page 94) or store-bought dairy-free milk

2 tablespoons raw cacao butter, preferably flavorless, melted

1 tablespoon avocado oil

½ teaspoon sunflower lecithin

Pinch of salt

In a high-speed blender, combine the coconut oil, cashew milk, cacao butter, oil, lecithin, and salt. Blend on high speed for 1 minute, until smooth. Transfer to an 8-ounce resealable container and freeze until firm, about 30 minutes.

STORAGE: The butter will keep refrigerated in an airtight container for up to 1 month.

MIX IT UP: To add flavor to 1 cup of the butter, mix in chopped fresh herbs (about ½ cup herbs) or add a pinch of Old Bay seasoning; sweeten the butter with ¼ teaspoon cinnamon sugar; or add tartness with 4 teaspoons grated orange zest.

Per Serving (1 teaspoon): Calories: 17; Total fat: 2g; Carbohydrates: 0g; Cholesterol: 0mg; Fiber: 0g; Protein: 0g; Sugar: 0g

96

Goat Cheese

Makes about 2 cups

This make-ahead recipe is great for entertaining. Probiotic powder, which you can find at any supermarket or drugstore, gives this cheese a nice tang and texture reminiscent of its goat's milk counterpart. Spread a little on the Mushroom Veggie Burgers (page 138) for extra decadence.

PREP TIME: 15 minutes, plus 20 hours to soak, drain, and chill

1 cup raw macadamia nuts, soaked in water for at least 4 hours or overnight, then rinsed and drained

1 cup raw cashews, soaked in water for at least 4 hours or overnight, then rinsed and drained

½ cup water

2 teaspoons freshly squeezed lemon juice

1 teaspoon dairy-free probiotic powder

1¼ teaspoons salt, divided

⅓ cup finely chopped fresh herbs, such as rosemary, parsley, and thyme

1 tablespoon grated lemon zest

½ teaspoon coarsely cracked black peppercorns

1. Place a strainer over a bowl and line the strainer with damp cheesecloth.

2. In a high-speed blender, combine the macadamia nuts, cashews, water, lemon juice, probiotic powder, and 1 teaspoon salt. Blend on high speed for about 1 minute, until smooth. Transfer the mixture to the strainer and fold over the sides of the cheesecloth to cover the cheese loosely. Place a weight on top, such as a heavy plate, and let drain at room temperature for at least 8 hours or overnight.

3. Lay a 12-inch square piece of plastic wrap on a work surface. Place the cheese in the middle and roll it into a log using the plastic wrap, then twist the ends to seal. Refrigerate for at least 8 hours, until set.

Continues →

97

4. In a small bowl, stir together the herbs, lemon zest, peppercorns, and remaining ¼ teaspoon salt. Spread the herbs on a plate, unwrap the cheese, and then roll the cheese log in the herb mixture to coat completely.

> **STORAGE:** Refrigerate the goat cheese in an airtight container for up to 1 week.
>
> **MIX IT UP:** Swap your favorite spices or dried herb blend for the fresh herbs and lemon peel, or use spiced roasted chopped nuts to coat the log instead.

Per Serving (2 tablespoons): Calories: 112; Total fat: 10g; Carbohydrates: 4g; Cholesterol: 0mg; Fiber: 1g; Protein: 2g; Sugar: 0g

Grated Parmesan Cheese

Makes about 1 cup

Parmesan in 1 minute? Yup—a few whirls in your food processor and you're ready to top your plate of pasta. I use nutritional yeast, a fiber-packed inactive yeast you can find in your local health food store, because it delivers a cheesy flavor. Macadamia nuts provide the full-fat richness here.

PREP TIME: 5 minutes

¾ cup raw macadamia nuts
¼ cup nutritional yeast
½ teaspoon salt

In a food processor or blender, combine the macadamia nuts, nutritional yeast, and salt. Pulse until the mixture resembles grated parmesan cheese.

STORAGE: Refrigerate the parmesan in a resealable container for up to 1 week.

SUBSTITUTION TIP: If you can't find macadamia nuts, use raw cashews.

99

Per Serving (¼ cup) Calories: 183; Total fat: 19g; Carbohydrates: 4g; Cholesterol: 0mg; Fiber: 2g; Protein: 3g; Sugar: 1g

Ricotta
Makes about 2 cups

When I set out to make ricotta without traditional ingredients like sheep's milk or cow's milk, what immediately came to mind were pine nuts. Indeed, the flavor of pine nuts reminds me of ricotta's Italian origins. A squeeze of lemon juice gives this ricotta its nice tang. Dollop it over Chicken Pasta with Creamy Vodka Sauce (page 143), Supreme Pizza Pasta Bake (page 38), or any of your favorite pasta recipes—about ¼ cup per serving.

PREP TIME: 5 minutes, plus 4 hours to soak

1 cup raw pine nuts, soaked in water for at least 4 hours or overnight, then rinsed and drained

1 cup raw macadamia nuts, soaked in water for at least 4 hours or overnight, then rinsed and drained

2 tablespoons olive oil

1 tablespoon freshly squeezed lemon juice

1 teaspoon salt

½ teaspoon date syrup

¼ cup plus 1 tablespoon water

1. In a food processor, combine the pine nuts, macadamia nuts, olive oil, lemon juice, salt, and date syrup. Pulse to combine.

2. With the motor running, slowly stream in the water, stopping to scrape down the sides of the bowl as needed. Process for about 3 minutes, until light and fluffy.

> **STORAGE:** Refrigerate the ricotta in an airtight container for up to 1 week.
>
> **INGREDIENT TIP:** Make sweet ricotta, which is great for spreading on toast or enjoying with a spoon. Use a neutral-flavored oil such as avocado oil instead of the olive oil and add 3 tablespoons sugar, 1 teaspoon vanilla, and the grated zest of 1 orange (optional).

Per Serving (¼ cup): Calories: 201; Total fat: 21g; Carbohydrates: 3g; Cholesterol: 0mg; Fiber: 2g; Protein: 2g; Sugar: 1g

100

Dairy-Free Cream Cheese

Makes about 1 cup

In my kitchen, I use cream cheese for both sweet and savory dishes, so I knew I had to develop a dairy-free knockoff that's thick and spreadable, just like the cream cheese you'd find in your supermarket's refrigerated case. You're welcome.

PREP TIME: 5 minutes, plus 5 hours to soak and chill

½ cup raw macadamia nuts, soaked in water for at least 4 hours or overnight, then rinsed and drained

½ cup raw cashews, soaked in water for at least 4 hours or overnight, then rinsed and drained

¼ cup refined coconut oil, melted

½ teaspoon dairy-free probiotic powder

½ teaspoon date syrup

¼ teaspoon salt

1. Place a strainer over a bowl and line the strainer with damp cheesecloth.

2. In a high-speed blender, combine the macadamia nuts, cashews, coconut oil, probiotic powder, date syrup, and salt. Blend on high speed for about 1 minute, until smooth.

3. Transfer the mixture to the cheesecloth-lined strainer and fold over the sides of the cheesecloth to cover the cheese loosely. Refrigerate for at least 1 hour to set.

STORAGE: Refrigerate the cream cheese in an airtight container for up to 1 week.

MIX IT UP: Flavor your cream cheese by stirring in chopped scallions, chopped sun-dried tomatoes, pickled jalapeños, or even chopped walnuts and soaked and drained raisins.

Per Serving (1 tablespoon): Calories 114 Total Fat 11g Carbohydrates 3g Cholesterol 0mg Fiber 1g Protein 2g Sugar 0g

Dairy-Free Sour Cream

Makes about 1 cup

I've added several layers of acidity here, including lemon juice, vinegar, and a dairy-free probiotic powder, to get the perfect sourness in this recipe. You can use this sour cream in both sweet and savory recipes. The longer you soak the nuts, the smoother the sour cream will be. If you can't find chickpea miso at your health food store, use a traditional soy-based miso.

PREP TIME: 6 minutes, plus 5 hours to soak and chill

1 cup raw cashews, soaked in water for at least 4 hours or overnight, then rinsed and drained

3 tablespoons freshly squeezed lemon juice

1 teaspoon distilled white vinegar

1 teaspoon gluten-free chickpea miso or soy-based miso

¾ teaspoon salt

½ teaspoon dairy-free probiotic powder

¾ cup water

In a high-speed blender, combine the cashews, lemon juice, vinegar, miso, salt, probiotic powder, and water. Blend on high speed for about 1 minute, until smooth. Refrigerate for about 1 hour until cold and thickened.

STORAGE: Refrigerate the sour cream in an airtight container for up to 1 week.

MIX IT UP: To use as a spicy dip, stir in some chopped chipotle chile in adobo sauce to taste.

Per Serving (2 tablespoons): Calories: 105; Total fat: 8g; Carbohydrates: 5g; Cholesterol: 0mg; Fiber: 1g; Protein: 3g; Sugar: 0g

102

White Cream Sauce

Makes 1½ cups

My mother taught me how to make a classic milk-based French white cream sauce, also called béchamel sauce, when I was a kid. It was the secret to her famous eggplant lasagna. Béchamel gives any recipe body and richness. Depending on your needs, you can thin this dairy- and gluten-free version and stir it into soups, use it as a base for macaroni and cheese, or layer it in your lasagna for a super-decadent meal.

PREP TIME: 5 minutes

COOK TIME: 12 minutes

2 tablespoons olive oil, Dairy-Free Butter (page 96), or store-bought dairy-free butter, melted

2 tablespoons gluten-free flour

1½ cups Cashew Milk (page 94) or store-bought dairy-free milk

1 teaspoon salt

¼ teaspoon ground nutmeg

1. In a small saucepan over medium heat, heat the olive oil. Whisk in the flour until smooth.

2. Slowly whisk in the milk and cook, whisking, for about 10 minutes, until thickened. Season with the salt and nutmeg, whisking to blend.

103

STORAGE: Refrigerate the sauce in an airtight container for up to 5 days.

INGREDIENT TIP: If you love garlic and want to flavor this creamy sauce even more, sauté 2 finely chopped garlic cloves in the olive oil for about 1 minute, until golden, before adding the flour and milk.

Per Serving (2 tablespoons): Calories: 23; Total fat: 3g; Carbohydrates: 0g; Cholesterol: 0mg; Fiber: 0g; Protein: 0g; Sugar: 0g

Cheese Sauce

Makes 2 cups

This versatile sauce is made with neutral-flavored cashews and nutritional yeast, a deactivated yeast with a salty, cheesy flavor. The red bell pepper lends flavor and gives the sauce its cheddar-like color.

PREP TIME: 20 minutes

2 cups raw cashews, soaked in hot water
   for 15 minutes, then rinsed and drained
½ cup chopped seeded red bell pepper
1 garlic clove, finely chopped
½ cup avocado oil
2 tablespoons nutritional yeast
1 tablespoon freshly squeezed lemon juice
2 teaspoons salt
½ cup water, plus more as needed

In a high-speed blender or food processor, combine the cashews, bell pepper, garlic, oil, nutritional yeast, lemon juice, salt, and ½ cup water. Process for about 2 minutes, until smooth, stopping to scrape down the sides as needed. If the consistency is too thick, add more water, 1 tablespoon at a time, blending until creamy.

STORAGE: Refrigerate the cheese sauce in an airtight container for up to 1 week.

MIX IT UP: Heat things up by adding 1 seeded and chopped jalapeño along with the other ingredients before processing.

Per Serving (2 tablespoons): Calories: 171; Total fat: 15g; Carbohydrates: 6g; Cholesterol: 0mg; Fiber: 1g; Protein: 4g; Sugar: 0g

104

Green Goddess Dressing

Makes about 2 cups

This is my go-to dressing, especially in summer. It's herb-flecked
and creamy, thanks to the avocado, and wonderfully refreshing
with its citrus juices.

PREP TIME: 10 minutes

1 garlic clove, peeled

1 tablespoon apple cider vinegar

1 tablespoon freshly squeezed lime juice

1 tablespoon freshly squeezed lemon juice

½ cup plus 2 tablespoons fresh cilantro
    leaves, divided

½ cup fresh basil leaves

½ cup fresh mint leaves

1 avocado, halved and pitted

¼ cup plus 2 tablespoons avocado oil

½ cup water, as needed

In a high-speed blender, combine the
garlic, vinegar, lime juice, lemon juice,
½ cup cilantro, the basil, mint, avocado
and avocado oil, and as much water as
needed to reach your desired consistency (see tip). Blend until smooth.
Add the remaining 2 tablespoons
cilantro and blend until chopped but
still visible.

STORAGE: Refrigerate the dressing in
an airtight container for up to 1 week.

INGREDIENT TIP: The consistency
of this dressing should depend on how
you will be using it. Add less water if
you want it thick and rich; add all the
water if you're using the dressing to coat
ingredients, such as in a potato salad.

Per Serving (2 tablespoons): Calories 67 Total fat 7g
Carbohydrates 2g Cholesterol 0mg Fiber 1g Protein
0g Sugar 0g

105

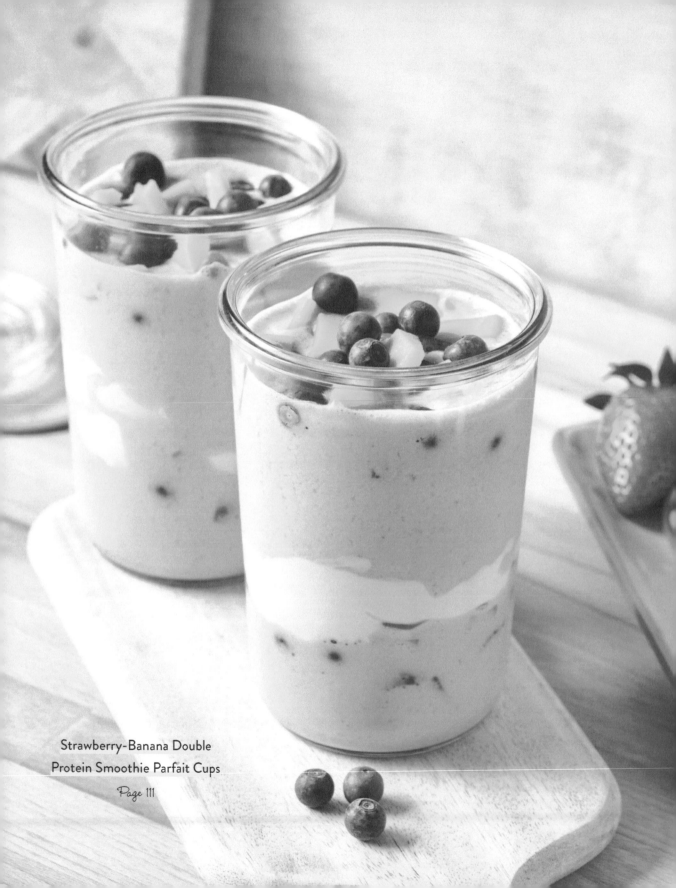

Strawberry-Banana Double
Protein Smoothie Parfait Cups

Page 111

Chapter Seven

BREAKFASTS

❋ ❋ ❋

Black Forest Energy Smoothie

Makes 4 smoothies

The flavor combination of chocolate and cherry is a longtime favorite of mine. I use protein powder in this smoothie, but you can swap in whatever nut butter you have in your pantry, if you prefer.

PREP TIME: 10 minutes

4 cups Cashew Milk (page 94) or store-bought unsweetened dairy-free milk

2 small bananas, cut into 1-inch pieces and frozen

2 cups frozen pitted cherries

½ cup unsweetened dairy-free protein powder

½ cup cacao powder or dairy-free unsweetened cocoa powder

1 teaspoon vanilla extract

4 teaspoons pure maple syrup (optional)

In a high-speed blender, combine the milk, bananas, cherries, protein powder, cacao powder, vanilla, and maple syrup (if using). Blend on high speed until smooth. (If your blender can't hold all the mixture, process in two batches.)

STORAGE: Place the blended smoothies in 4 resealable containers. Cover, label, and refrigerate for up to 2 days. Or, portion one-fourth of each ingredient into each of 4 resealable freezer-safe containers, cover, label, and freeze for up to 1 month.

TO SERVE: Shake the contents of 1 refrigerated container well. Or, transfer the contents of 1 frozen container to a blender and blend as directed.

INGREDIENT TIP: If you're not a chocolate lover, omit the cacao powder for a cherry-vanilla smoothie.

Per Serving (1 smoothie): Calories: 349; Total fat: 10g; Carbohydrates: 49g; Cholesterol: 0mg; Fiber: 14g; Protein: 32g; Sugar: 23g

108

Pumpkin Spice Breakfast Smoothie

Makes 4 smoothies

My favorite time of year to make this smoothie is the holiday season, when nearly everything is flavored with pumpkin spice. I add flaxseed oil here, an antioxidant rich in omega-3 fatty acids, not just for the health benefits but also as an emulsifier to make the smoothie extra creamy. Look for a pumpkin pie spice blend made with cinnamon, ginger, cloves, and nutmeg at your local supermarket.

PREP TIME: 10 minutes

2 cups pumpkin purée

3 cups Cashew Milk (page 94) or store-bought unsweetened dairy-free milk

¼ cup flaxseed oil

½ cup almond flour

2 bananas, cut into 1-inch pieces and frozen

4 teaspoons pumpkin pie spice, plus more for sprinkling

In a high-speed blender, combine the pumpkin, milk, flaxseed oil, almond flour, bananas, and pumpkin pie spice. Blend on high speed until smooth.

STORAGE: Place the blended smoothies in 4 resealable containers. Cover, label, and refrigerate for up to 2 days. Or, portion one-fourth of each ingredient into each of 4 resealable freezer-safe containers, cover, label, and freeze for up to 1 month.

TO SERVE: Shake the contents of 1 refrigerated container well. Or, transfer the contents of 1 frozen container to a blender and blend as directed. Sprinkle with pumpkin pie spice.

SUBSTITUTION TIP: No almond flour or almonds? Use almond butter or peanut butter instead.

Per Serving (1 smoothie): Calories 311; Total fat 20g; Carbohydrates 32g; Cholesterol 0mg; Fiber 6g; Protein 4g; Sugar 17g

Super Greens Smoothie Bowl

Makes 4 smoothie bowls

Packed with superfoods such as avocado, spinach, ginger, and a bit of caffeine from the energizing matcha powder, this creamy green smoothie bowl makes a satisfying breakfast that will leave you feeling full for hours. Finish it with plenty of fresh berries and crunchy nuts, and your day will be off to an incredible start. Look for matcha powder in the tea section of your local supermarket.

PREP TIME: 10 minutes

4 cups Cashew Milk (page 94) or store-bought unsweetened dairy-free milk

½ cup unsweetened dairy-free protein powder

2 bananas, cut into 1-inch pieces and frozen

2 cups baby spinach

1 avocado, halved and pitted

4 teaspoons matcha powder

4 teaspoons chopped peeled fresh ginger

4 teaspoons pure maple syrup (optional)

Unsweetened shredded coconut, for topping (optional)

Chopped nuts, for topping (optional)

Fresh berries, for topping (optional)

In a high-speed blender, combine the milk, protein powder, bananas, spinach, avocado flesh, matcha, ginger, and maple syrup (if using). Blend on high speed until smooth.

STORAGE: Place the blended smoothies in 4 resealable containers. Cover, label, and refrigerate for up to 2 days. Or, portion one-fourth of each ingredient into each of 4 resealable freezer-safe containers, cover, label, and freeze for up to 1 month.

TO SERVE: Shake the contents of 1 refrigerated container well. Or, transfer the contents of 1 frozen container to a blender and blend as directed. Sprinkle with toppings, if desired.

INGREDIENT TIP: If you're not a fan of protein powder, leave it out.

Per Serving (1 smoothie bowl): Calories: 328; Total fat: 10g; Carbohydrates: 41g; Cholesterol: 0mg; Fiber: 7g; Protein: 22g; Sugar: 23g

110

Strawberry-Banana Double Protein Smoothie Parfait Cups

Makes 4 parfait cups

Not only are parfaits pretty, but they are also easy to make ahead so you have them ready in the morning. Here, I layer a strawberry-banana smoothie with dairy-free yogurt and chopped fresh seasonal fruit.

PREP TIME: 15 minutes

4 bananas, cut into 1-inch pieces
  and frozen
2 cups frozen hulled strawberries
½ cup unsweetened dairy-free
  protein powder
2 cups plain dairy-free yogurt, divided
4 cups Cashew Milk (page 94)
  or store-bought unsweetened
  dairy-free milk
4 teaspoons pure maple syrup (optional)
Salt (optional)
1 cup chopped fresh seasonal fruit, such as
  strawberries, blueberries, or mango, plus
  more for topping

In a high-speed blender, combine the banana, strawberries, protein powder, 1 cup of the yogurt, the milk, maple syrup (if using), and a pinch of salt (if using). Blend on high speed until smooth.

STORAGE: In each of 4 (16-ounce) glass jars with lids or travel mugs, layer ¼ cup of the blended smoothie, ¼ cup of the chopped fruit, and ¼ cup of the remaining yogurt. Evenly divide the remaining smoothie among the cups and top each with more fruit. Seal the lids. Label and refrigerate the smoothies in the sealed glass jars for up to 2 days.

TO SERVE: Shake the contents of 1 refrigerated jar well.

MIX IT UP: If you're feeling indulgent, add some dairy-free chocolate chips to the mix.

111

Per Serving (1 parfait cup): Calories 357; Total fat 6g; Carbohydrates 62g; Cholesterol 0mg; Fiber 6g; Protein 14g; Sugar 37g

Chocolate Chunk Protein Muffins

Makes 12 muffins

This is the easiest—and tastiest—way to get a boost of protein and energy into your day. The morning rush comes from the almond flour and collagen peptides. Collagen peptides are a protein powerhouse that help promote skin and hair health while reducing inflammation. These muffins are great to enjoy on the go, and they make a great snack option.

PREP TIME: 15 minutes

COOK TIME: 20 minutes

½ cup Cashew Milk (page 94) or store-bought unsweetened dairy-free milk

½ teaspoon apple cider vinegar

1 cup almond flour

¼ cup collagen peptides or unsweetened dairy-free protein powder (optional)

⅔ cup unsweetened cocoa powder

1 cup sugar

1 teaspoon baking powder

1 teaspoon baking soda

½ teaspoon salt

½ cup avocado oil

2 large eggs

2 teaspoons vanilla extract

1 cup coarsely chopped dark (70%) chocolate

1. Preheat the oven to 375°F. Line a standard 12-cup muffin pan with paper liners.

2. In a small bowl, whisk together the milk and vinegar.

3. In a large bowl, whisk the almond flour, collagen peptides (if using), cocoa powder, sugar, baking powder, baking soda, and salt to combine.

4. In a medium bowl, whisk the avocado oil, eggs, vanilla, and the milk mixture. Stir the wet ingredients into the dry ingredients until just combined. Stir in the chocolate. Pour the batter into the muffin pan, filling each cup about two-thirds full.

5. Bake for about 20 minutes, until springy to the touch and a toothpick inserted into the center of a muffin comes out clean. Let cool in the pan set on a wire rack, then remove the muffins from the pan.

STORAGE: Place the muffins in a large resealable container. Cover, label, and refrigerate for up to 5 days, or freeze for up to 1 month.

TO SERVE: Enjoy the muffin from the refrigerator. Or, if frozen, let the muffin sit overnight at room temperature to thaw, or place the muffin on a paper towel and microwave on high power for about 30 seconds.

SUBSTITUTION TIP: Want to make these healthier? Swap in granulated maple sugar for the granulated sugar. High in antioxidants, unrefined maple sugar has a lower glycemic index than conventional granulated sugar, which means you won't get a sugar rush.

Per Serving (1 muffin): Calories: 279; Total fat: 19g; Carbohydrates: 27g; Cholesterol: 31mg; Fiber: 3g; Protein: 4g; Sugar: 21g

Lemon-Poppy Seed Buttermilk Waffles
Makes 4 servings

Dairy-free buttermilk gives these waffles a lovely airiness and slight sour taste. Chia seeds, though optional, add a bit of crunch and some healthy fiber, along with the poppy seeds. If you run out of time on meal-prep day, this batter gets even better after it sits overnight in the fridge. Just let it come to room temperature before cooking.

PREP TIME: 10 minutes

COOK TIME: 5 minutes

1½ cups Cashew Milk (page 94) or store-bought unsweetened dairy-free milk

1½ teaspoons apple cider vinegar

1½ cups gluten-free flour

2 tablespoons sugar

2 teaspoons baking powder

½ teaspoon baking soda

½ teaspoon salt

⅓ cup avocado oil

2 large eggs, at room temperature

2 teaspoons vanilla extract

Grated zest of 2 lemons

2 tablespoons freshly squeezed lemon juice

2 tablespoons chia seeds (optional)

1 tablespoon poppy seeds

Nonstick cooking spray

Pure maple syrup, warmed, for serving (optional)

1. In a small bowl, stir together the milk and vinegar.

2. In a large bowl, whisk the flour, sugar, baking powder, baking soda, and salt to combine.

3. Preheat a waffle iron to medium-high according to the manufacturer's directions.

4. In a medium bowl, whisk the milk mixture, avocado oil, eggs, vanilla, lemon zest, lemon juice, chia seeds (if using), and poppy seeds until blended. Stir the wet ingredients into the dry ingredients. Whisk to combine.

5. Coat the waffle iron with cooking spray. Pour about ⅓ cup of batter into each waffle iron section. Close and cook for about 5 minutes, until crisp. Continue to make the waffles until the batter is used up.

114

STORAGE: Place the waffles in 4 individual resealable containers. Cover, label, and refrigerate for up to 5 days, or freeze for up to 1 month.

REHEAT FROM THE FRIDGE: Place the waffle on a paper towel and microwave on high power for about 30 seconds. If you prefer a crisper waffle, heat it in a toaster oven on the lightest or lowest heat setting for about 90 seconds if refrigerated and for up to 3 minutes if frozen, until crisp. To heat the maple syrup, if desired, place it in a microwave-safe container and heat on high power for about 15 seconds, until warmed.

MIX IT UP: For a fruitier variation, add a handful of fresh blueberries to the batter before making the waffles.

Per Serving (1 waffle): Calories: 421; Total fat: 24g; Carbohydrates: 45g; Cholesterol: 93mg; Fiber: 5g; Protein: 8g; Sugar: 10g

Baked Eggs with Sweet Potatoes, Kale, and Parm

Makes 4 servings

I first had baked eggs in a tiny restaurant in Upstate New York. I couldn't believe how flavorful they were. I also like how flexible this recipe is—you can add your favorite ingredients or leftovers to the eggs before baking. In this recipe, I use a hearty combination of sweet potatoes, mushrooms, kale, and parmesan for a breakfast or brunch that'll keep you satisfied for hours.

PREP TIME: 15 minutes

COOK TIME: 30 minutes

1 (10-ounce) package button mushrooms, trimmed and coarsely chopped

1 large sweet potato, peeled and coarsely chopped

1 small onion, coarsely chopped

3½ tablespoons olive oil, divided

Salt

Freshly ground black pepper

4 ounces fresh kale, preferably lacinato, ribs trimmed away and leafy portions chopped

⅓ cup water

½ garlic clove

Nonstick cooking spray

8 large eggs

Grated Parmesan Cheese (page 99) or store-bought dairy-free grated parmesan-style cheese, for sprinkling

1. Preheat the oven to 450°F. Have ready a bowl of ice water.

2. On a baking sheet, toss together the mushrooms, sweet potato, onion, and 2 tablespoons of the olive oil to coat everything well. Generously season with salt and pepper.

3. Roast for about 20 minutes, until the vegetables are tender and golden. Transfer to a bowl.

4. Bring a large pot of salted water to a boil over high heat. Add the kale and blanch for 10 seconds. Drain and shock in the ice water to stop the cooking. Squeeze dry.

5. Transfer the kale to a food processor. Add the remaining 1½ tablespoons olive oil, the water, and garlic. Process until smooth. Season with ½ teaspoon salt.

6. Preheat the broiler and place an oven rack 10 inches from the heat source.

7. Place 4 (1-cup) oven-safe baking dishes on the baking sheet, and generously coat each with cooking spray. Crack 2 eggs into each dish.

Scatter some of the sweet potato hash over each cup and drizzle with some of the kale. Sprinkle the parmesan on top.

8. Broil for 6 to 8 minutes, until the egg whites are set and the yolks are still a bit runny.

STORAGE: Let cool, cover the dishes, label, and refrigerate for up to 5 days.

REHEAT FROM THE FRIDGE: Warm the baking dish in a preheated 350°F toaster oven for about 10 minutes, or transfer to a microwave-safe container and cover with plastic wrap, leaving one end open for steam to escape. Microwave on high power for about 1 minute, until heated through.

MIX IT UP: Swap in cherry tomatoes, corn, and spinach for the mushrooms, sweet potato, and kale.

117

Per Serving: Calories 336; Total fat 24g; Carbohydrates 15g; Cholesterol 377mg; Fiber 3g; Protein 19g; Sugar 4g

Chicken Carnitas Tacos with Scrambled Eggs and Chipotle Cranberry Sauce

Makes 4 tacos

The beauty of breakfast tacos is that you can add almost any ingredient to the scrambled egg filling and, likely, they'll turn out beautifully. Originally, I developed this recipe to use leftover turkey from Thanksgiving. Since I don't often have extra roasted turkey on hand, I now mostly use cooked chicken.

PREP TIME: 15 minutes
COOK TIME: 15 minutes

4 large eggs

¼ teaspoon salt

¼ teaspoon freshly ground black pepper

2 tablespoons avocado oil, divided

2 cups shredded rotisserie chicken

1 cup cranberry sauce

2 canned chipotle chiles in adobo sauce, chopped

2 avocados, peeled, halved, pitted, and cut lengthwise into slices

Chopped fresh cilantro, for topping

4 (6-inch) corn tortillas

1. In a medium bowl, whisk the eggs while adding the salt and pepper.

2. In a large nonstick skillet over medium-high heat, heat 1 tablespoon of the avocado oil. Add the eggs and cook, stirring, for 2 to 3 minutes, until set but still soft.

3. Preheat the broiler.

4. On a rimmed baking sheet, toss together the shredded chicken and remaining 1 tablespoon avocado oil. Broil for about 5 minutes, turning occasionally, until browned and crisp.

5. In a small saucepan over medium heat, stir together the cranberry sauce and chipotle chiles. Cook for about 5 minutes, until warmed through.

118

STORAGE: Let cool. Place each of the following in 4 separate resealable containers (making 24 total): the scrambled eggs, chicken, sauce, avocado, cilantro, and tortillas. Cover, label, and refrigerate for up to 5 days.

REHEAT FROM THE FRIDGE: Wrap the tortilla in a damp paper towel and microwave on high power for 30 seconds to 1 minute. To serve, spread the sauce on the warmed tortilla and top with the chicken, scrambled eggs, and the cilantro. Fold in half and microwave on a microwave-safe plate on high power for about 30 seconds, until heated through. Serve with the avocado.

INGREDIENT TIP: I love the extra heat the chipotle chiles add to the sweet-tart cranberry sauce, but if you don't, then leave them out.

Per Serving (1 taco): Calories: 464; Total fat: 28g; Carbohydrates: 26g; Cholesterol: 240mg; Fiber: 8g; Protein: 30g; Sugar: 6g

Breakfast Pizza Frittata

Makes 4 servings

I grew up in an Italian household, and my mom used to turn our leftovers into frittatas—think spaghetti, chili, and cheese. Here, I turn a classic Margherita pizza into a frittata by combining my instant pizza sauce, pepperoni, dairy-free mozzarella, and fresh basil.

PREP TIME: 15 minutes

COOK TIME: 40 minutes

12 large eggs

1 cup cashew cream (see Cashew Milk tip, page 94) or store-bought dairy-free heavy cream

½ cup Grated Parmesan Cheese (page 99) or store-bought dairy-free parmesan-style cheese

Salt

Freshly ground black pepper

4 tablespoons olive oil, divided

4 ounces pepperoni, finely chopped (about 1 cup)

3 tablespoons finely chopped onion

2 garlic cloves, chopped

1 cup canned crushed tomatoes

6 ounces shredded dairy-free mozzarella-style cheese (about 1½ cups)

Fresh basil leaves, for topping

1. Preheat the oven to 400°F.

2. In a large bowl, whisk the eggs, cashew cream, and parmesan until blended. Season with salt and pepper and whisk to combine.

3. In a large ovenproof skillet over medium-high heat, heat 2 tablespoons of the olive oil. Add the egg mixture and cook, without stirring, for about 5 minutes, until the edges begin to set. Transfer the skillet to the oven and bake for about 10 minutes, until golden but the eggs are not completely set.

4. Meanwhile, in another skillet over medium-high heat, heat the remaining 2 tablespoons olive oil. Add the pepperoni, onion, and garlic. Cook about 3 minutes, stirring occasionally.

5. Stir in the tomatoes. Bring to a simmer and cook for about 8 minutes, until thickened.

120

6. Remove the frittata from the oven and top with the tomato sauce and the mozzarella. Return the skillet to the oven and cook for about 10 minutes more, until the center is set and the cheese is melted.

STORAGE: Cool the frittata and cut it into 4 portions, then place each in a resealable container. Cover, label, and refrigerate for up to 5 days, or freeze for up to 1 month. Wrap the basil leaves in 4 portions, each in a damp paper towel, then label and refrigerate for up to 5 days.

REHEAT FROM THE FRIDGE: Transfer to a microwave-safe container and heat on low power for about 30 seconds, until warm. To serve, top with the basil leaves.

REHEAT FROM THE FREEZER: Thaw in the fridge overnight. Reheat as from the fridge.

SUBSTITUTION TIP: Want to make this vegetarian? Omit the pepperoni.

Per Serving Calories: 760 Total fat: 62g Carbohydrates: 20g Cholesterol: 598mg Fiber: 4g Protein: 33g Sugar: 8g

Hash Brown Waffles with Breakfast Sausage and Fried Eggs

Makes 4 servings

I have an obsession with waffles; I try to cook almost anything in a waffle maker, including grilled cheese, pizza, quesadillas, and even brownies! Here is an example: sausage and eggs with crispy hash brown waffles in place of the classic home fries.

PREP TIME: 15 minutes

COOK TIME: 25 minutes

3 tablespoons avocado oil, divided
8 precooked breakfast sausages
3 Yukon Gold potatoes (about 1½ pounds), peeled, grated, and squeezed dry
½ onion, grated
¾ teaspoon salt, plus more for seasoning
Nonstick cooking spray
4 large eggs, at room temperature
Freshly ground black pepper

1. In a large nonstick skillet over medium heat, heat 1 tablespoon of the avocado oil. Add the sausages and cook for about 3 minutes per side, until browned and heated through.

2. In a small bowl, stir together the potatoes, onion, 1 tablespoon of the avocado oil, and the salt.

3. Preheat a waffle iron (see tip) to medium-high heat according to the manufacturer's instructions and coat it with cooking spray. Place about ½ cup of the potato mixture into each waffle section. Close the waffle iron and cook for about 10 minutes, until golden and crisp.

4. Meanwhile, in a large skillet over medium heat, heat the remaining 1 tablespoon avocado oil. Crack the eggs into the skillet and season with salt and pepper. Cook, turning once, for about 3 minutes, until the whites are set and the yolks are still slightly runny.

122

STORAGE: Place each of the following in 4 separate resealable containers (making 12 total): the waffles, sausages, and eggs separately in 12 resealable containers for up to 5 days. Cover, label, and refrigerate.

REHEAT FROM THE FRIDGE: To reheat the eggs, transfer the egg to a microwave-safe container and microwave on medium power for about 30 seconds until warmed through. To reheat the sausages, place 2 on a microwave-safe plate and cover with a paper towel. Microwave on high power for about 45 seconds, until heated through. To reheat the waffles, place a waffle on a paper towel and microwave on high power for about 30 seconds. If you prefer a crisper waffle, heat it in a toaster oven on the lightest or lowest heat setting for about 90 seconds, until crisp. To serve, place the waffle on a plate and top with 2 sausages and 1 fried egg.

COOKING TIP: No waffle maker? No problem. Cook the grated potato mixture in a greased skillet over medium-high heat. Using a spatula, press the mixture into an even layer. Cook for about 5 minutes, flipping once halfway through the cooking time, until golden and crispy.

Per Serving: Calories: 448; Total fat: 26g; Carbohydrates: 29g; Cholesterol: 186mg; Fiber: 4g; Protein: 26g; Sugar: 3g

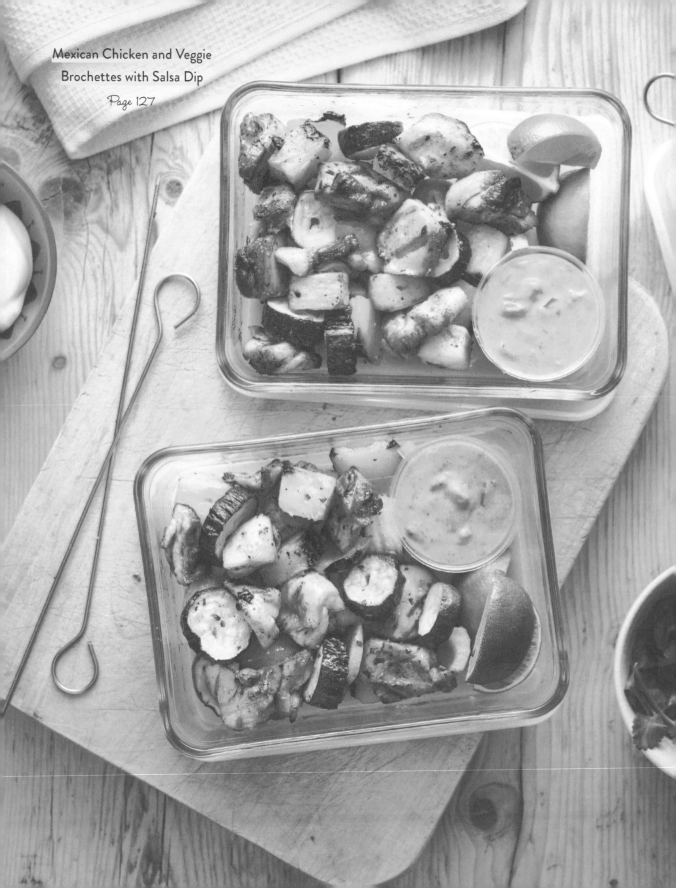

Mexican Chicken and Veggie
Brochettes with Salsa Dip

Page 127

Chapter Eight

LUNCHES AND DINNERS

✳ ✳ ✳

Crispy Baked Fish Sticks
Makes 4 servings

Fish sticks remind me of my childhood. My mother was a stay-at-home mom who cooked every meal from scratch. When my father would travel for work, she'd give herself a much-deserved break and make my brother and me frozen foods for dinner, which we loved. These days, I like to make homemade knockoffs of my favorite frozen foods, including these fish sticks.

PREP TIME: 15 minutes

COOK TIME: 25 minutes

Nonstick cooking spray
1 cup crushed gluten-free rice cereal
½ cup grits
1 tablespoon paprika
1 teaspoon garlic powder
½ teaspoon salt
1 large egg white
1 tablespoon water
1½ pounds cod or tilapia fillets, cut into ¾-by-4-inch strips, patted dry
4 lemon wedges

126

1. Preheat the oven to 400°F. Coat a baking sheet with cooking spray.

2. In a shallow dish, stir together the cereal crumbs, grits, paprika, garlic powder, and salt. In a second shallow dish, whisk the egg white and water.

3. Dredge the fish in the egg-white mixture, then coat completely with the crumb mixture. Place the coated fish on the prepared baking sheet.

4. Bake for about 25 minutes, until golden.

STORAGE: Let cool, then divide the fish among 4 small resealable containers and add 1 lemon wedge to each. Cover, label, and refrigerate for up to 3 days.

REHEAT FROM THE FRIDGE: Preheat a toaster oven or conventional oven to 350°F. Line a baking sheet with parchment paper and lay the fish sticks on the prepared sheet. Let the fish come to room temperature. Bake for about 15 minutes, until heated through. Microwave reheating is not recommended.

COOKING TIP: Want a fish fry? In a large skillet over medium-high heat, heat ½ cup avocado oil. Working in batches and adding ¼ cup oil between batches, cook the fish until golden brown and cooked through, about 3 minutes per side.

Per Serving: Calories: 171; Total fat: 2g; Carbohydrates: 7g; Cholesterol: 83mg; Fiber: 1g; Protein: 32g; Sugar: 1g

Mexican Chicken and Veggie Brochettes with Salsa Dip

Makes 4 servings

I love making these brochettes on my grill in the summer for garden parties and on Cinco de Mayo. If you're cooking with the kids, let them help you assemble the brochettes.

PREP TIME: 15 minutes

COOK TIME: 16 minutes

1¼ pounds boneless, skinless chicken thighs (about 8 thighs), cut into 1½-inch pieces

Olive oil, for drizzling

¼ cup finely chopped fresh cilantro

Salt

Freshly ground black pepper

1 bell pepper, any color, seeded and cut into 1½-inch pieces

6 ounces cubed fresh pineapple (about 1½ cups)

2 zucchini, cut into ½-inch-thick slices

1½ cups salsa of choice

¾ cup Dairy-Free Sour Cream (page 102) or store-bought dairy-free sour cream

4 lime wedges

1. Preheat a grill to medium heat (see tip).

2. Drizzle the chicken with some olive oil, sprinkle with cilantro, and generously season with salt and pepper.

3. Thread some skewers, alternating pieces of chicken, bell pepper, pineapple, and zucchini. Place the skewers on the grill and close the lid. Cook for 8 minutes. Turn the skewers, close the lid, and cook for about 8 minutes more, until the chicken is cooked through and the juices of the chicken run clear when pricked.

4. In a small bowl, stir together the salsa and sour cream. Season to taste with salt.

127

Continues →

STORAGE: Let cool, then remove the chicken and veggies from the skewers, if desired, and evenly divide among 4 medium resealable containers; add 1 lime wedge to each container. Cover, label, and refrigerate for up to 3 days. Divide the salsa mixture cream among 4 small resealable containers. Cover, label, and refrigerate for up to 3 days.

REHEAT FROM THE FRIDGE: Preheat the oven to 400°F. Line a baking sheet with parchment paper and place the brochettes, or the contents of the container if you've removed the food from the brochettes, on the prepared sheet. Bake for about 10 minutes, until heated through, turning once halfway through the cooking time. To reheat in the microwave, remove the food from the brochettes if not already done and place on a microwave-safe plate. Heat on high power for 2 minutes, turning the food once halfway through the cooking time.

COOKING TIP: You can also bake these in the oven. Preheat the oven to 425°F. Line a baking sheet with parchment paper and place a wire rack above it. Place the chicken skewers on the rack. Bake for about 20 minutes, turning once, until the chicken is cooked through and the juices run clear.

MIX IT UP: Swap in pieces of boneless, skinless chicken breast for the chicken thighs.

Per Serving: Calories: 355; Total fat: 18g; Carbohydrates: 20g; Cholesterol: 119mg; Fiber: 4g; Protein: 32g; Sugar: 13g

Chinese Orange Chicken with Broccoli Basmati

Makes 4 servings

I spent five years in San Francisco as a child, and going out to Chinese restaurants there was a regular occurrence. One of my favorite dishes was orange chicken, so I decided to make a version of the classic recipe at home.

PREP TIME: 15 minutes

COOK TIME: 35 minutes

FOR THE RICE

2 tablespoons avocado oil
1 small onion, finely chopped
3 cups chopped fresh broccoli florets
  (from about ½ head)
1½ cups basmati rice
¾ teaspoon salt
2½ cups water

FOR THE ORANGE CHICKEN

3 tablespoons ketchup
2 tablespoons tamari
1½ tablespoons rice wine vinegar
2 teaspoons finely chopped peeled
  fresh ginger
2 teaspoons finely chopped garlic
Grated zest of 1 orange
4 boneless, skinless chicken breasts (about
  2 pounds), cut into 1½-inch pieces
2 red bell peppers, seeded and cut into
  1-inch pieces

TO MAKE THE RICE

1. In a medium saucepan over medium heat, heat the avocado oil. Add the onion and cook for 3 minutes, stirring occasionally. Add the broccoli and cook for 3 minutes more.

2. Add the rice and cook, stirring, for 1 minute. Stir in the salt and water, increase the heat to high, and bring the rice to a boil. Cover the pan, reduce the heat to low, and simmer for about 15 minutes, until tender. Fluff with a fork.

TO MAKE THE ORANGE CHICKEN

3. While the rice cooks, in a medium bowl, whisk together the ketchup, tamari, vinegar, ginger, garlic, and orange zest. Add the chicken and toss to coat. Let marinate for 5 minutes.

4. Preheat a large skillet over medium-high heat. Add the chicken and marinade, as well as

129

Continues →

the red bell peppers. Cook for 8 to 10 minutes, stirring occasionally, until the chicken is cooked through.

STORAGE: Let cool, then evenly divide the chicken among 4 medium resealable containers; divide the rice among 4 small resealable containers. Cover, label, and refrigerate for up to 5 days.

REHEAT FROM THE FRIDGE: Place the chicken and rice in a microwave-safe dish and add 1 tablespoon water. Cover with a paper towel. Microwave on high power for about 2 minutes, until warmed through.

INGREDIENT TIP: As we use only the orange zest here, you can refrigerate the leftover orange for up to 2 days, but it will start to dry out without the peel. Squeeze the juice into seltzer for a refreshing spritzer.

MIX IT UP: Heat things up by adding some of your favorite hot sauce to the chicken.

Per Serving: Calories: 627; Total fat: 11g; Carbohydrates: 69g; Cholesterol: 130mg; Fiber: 4g; Protein: 60g; Sugar: 8g

Pressed Caesar Tuna Melts

Makes 4 melts

The tuna melt diner classic is easier to make than you think. Top it with Caesar dressing, and it takes on an extra-flavorful, creamy dimension. In keeping with the retro experience, serve a dill pickle alongside each melt. If you're gluten-free, just use your favorite gluten-free sliced bread and gluten-free Worcestershire sauce. If you have a panini press, here's your opportunity to use it; if not, you can cook them in a skillet.

PREP TIME: 10 minutes

COOK TIME: 3 minutes

FOR THE CAESAR DRESSING

¼ cup plus 2 tablespoons mayonnaise

¼ cup Grated Parmesan Cheese (page 99) or store-bought dairy-free parmesan-style cheese

¼ cup freshly squeezed lemon juice

¼ cup water

2 canned anchovy fillets

2 garlic cloves, peeled

2 teaspoons Worcestershire sauce

Salt

Freshly ground black pepper

FOR THE TUNA MELTS

2 (5-ounce) cans tuna, drained and flaked

½ cup shredded carrot (about 1 small carrot)

8 regular or gluten-free bread slices

4 slices dairy-free cheddar-style cheese

4 tomato slices

1 tablespoon Dairy-Free Butter (page 96) or store-bought dairy-free butter (optional)

TO MAKE THE CAESAR DRESSING

1. In a blender, combine the mayonnaise, parmesan, lemon juice, water, anchovies, garlic, and Worcestershire sauce. Blend until smooth, then season to taste with salt and pepper.

TO MAKE THE TUNA MELTS

2. In a medium bowl, stir together the tuna and carrot, then add the Caesar dressing and stir until well combined. Divide the tuna salad among 4 bread slices. Top each with a cheese slice and tomato slice, then top with the remaining 4 bread slices.

3. If using, preheat a panini press according to the manufacturer's instructions.

131

Continues →

4. Put the sandwiches on the panini press and close the lid. Cook for about
    3 minutes, until the cheese is melted. Alternatively, preheat a large skillet
    over medium heat and melt the butter. Add the sandwiches and cook for
    about 4 minutes per side or until the bread is golden brown and the cheese
    is melted.

STORAGE: Place each tuna melt in a resealable sandwich bag, seal, label, and refrigerate
for up to 5 days. Or, place each melt in a resealable freezer bag, seal, label, and freeze for up to
1 month.

REHEAT FROM THE FREEZER: Place the tuna melt on a microwave-safe plate and heat
on medium power for about 3 minutes, until thawed and heated through. To serve, cut the
melt in half.

COOKING TIP: Too fishy for you? Omit the anchovies from the Caesar dressing and season
to taste with salt.

Per Serving (1 melt): Calories: 468; Total fat: 25g; Carbohydrates: 36g; Cholesterol: 32mg; Fiber: 3g; Protein: 23g;
Sugar: 4g

Tahini Tuna Salad Stacks

Makes 4 servings

Since it's one of my favorite healthy convenience foods
for a quick lunch (or dinner), I've taken canned tuna—high in
protein and omega-3s—beyond the classic mayo-laced sandwich or
salad. Garlicky tahini is swapped for the standard mayonnaise,
which then takes canned tuna to the next level.

PREP TIME: 15 minutes

½ cup water

6 tablespoons tahini

2 tablespoons freshly squeezed lemon juice

2 garlic cloves, peeled

1 teaspoon ground cumin

2 (5-ounce) cans tuna, drained and flaked

2 tablespoons chopped fresh parsley, plus
   more for garnish

Salt

Freshly ground black pepper

2 large tomatoes, each cut into 4 slices

Sesame seeds, toasted, for garnish

1. In a blender or food processor, combine the water, tahini, lemon juice, garlic, and cumin. Blend until smooth. Transfer to a medium bowl.

2. Stir in the tuna and parsley. Taste and season with salt and pepper.

STORAGE: In each of 4 medium resealable containers, place 1 tomato slice. Top with one-eighth of the tuna, another tomato slice, and the remaining tuna. Sprinkle with a little more parsley and the sesame seeds. Cover the containers and refrigerate the stacks for up to 2 days.

MIX IT UP: Want more of a salad? Add some lightly dressed mixed salad greens to the stack, or top the mixed greens with the stack.

133

Per Serving: Calories 227; Total fat: 13g; Carbohydrates 9g; Cholesterol 19mg; Fiber 3g; Protein 20g; Sugar 3g

Polenta with Texas Turkey Ragù

Makes 4 servings

Italian and Tex-Mex flavors come together in this tasty, humble dish. Traditionally, ragù is a meat-based sauce commonly served with pasta. In this recipe, I swap out the pasta for polenta, an Italian-style cornmeal. I prefer using the coarse-ground polenta, which has a wonderfully toothsome texture but takes a while to cook. If you're short on time, use instant polenta, which cooks up in about 5 minutes.

PREP TIME: 15 minutes

COOK TIME: 55 minutes

3½ cups water

2 teaspoons salt, divided

1 cup coarse-ground polenta

2 tablespoons olive oil

2 garlic cloves, finely chopped

1 red onion, chopped

2 bell peppers, any color, chopped

1 pound ground turkey

1½ tablespoons regular or gluten-free chili powder

1 teaspoon unsweetened cocoa powder

1 teaspoon dried oregano

1 cinnamon stick

1 (15-ounce) can fire-roasted diced tomatoes, with juices

1 cup regular or gluten-free chicken broth

1 (15-ounce) can regular or gluten-free chickpeas, rinsed and drained

1 scallion, green and white parts sliced, for topping

1. In a medium saucepan over high heat, combine the water and 1 teaspoon salt. Bring to a boil. Slowly whisk in the polenta. Cover the pan, reduce the heat to medium, and cook for about 45 minutes, whisking often, until thickened.

2. Meanwhile, in a medium pot over medium heat, heat the olive oil. Add the garlic, red onion, and bell peppers. Cook about 7 minutes, stirring, until softened.

3. Increase the heat to medium-high and stir in the ground turkey. Cook, breaking up the meat with a spoon, for about 4 minutes, until cooked through and no longer pink.

4. Stir in the chili powder, cocoa powder, oregano, cinnamon stick, and remaining teaspoon salt.

5. Add the tomatoes and chicken broth. Bring to a boil. Reduce the heat to low and cover the pot. Simmer for 15 minutes.

6. Stir in the chickpeas and cook, uncovered, for about 10 minutes, until thickened slightly.

STORAGE: Gather 4 medium and 4 small resealable containers. Evenly divide the ragù among the medium containers and the polenta among the small containers. Cover, label, and refrigerate for up to 5 days. Place one-fourth of the scallion in each of 4 small resealable bags, seal, label, and refrigerate for up to 5 days.

REHEAT FROM THE FRIDGE: Place the polenta in a microwave-safe container and top with the ragù. Cover with a microwave-safe lid set askew, and microwave on high power for about 3 minutes until warmed through. Serve topped with the scallion.

INGREDIENT TIP: Swap in grits, made of a finer grind of white corn, for a heartier polenta.

Per Serving: Calories 404; Total fat 12g; Carbohydrates 42g; Cholesterol 62mg; Fiber 8g; Protein 36g; Sugar 8g

Sloppy Joe–Smothered Sweet Potato Fries

Makes 4 servings

When I started eating a grain-free Paleo diet, I developed this recipe, which is total comfort served on a plate—crispy roasted sweet potatoes covered with a chicken-based sloppy joe, a dish typically enjoyed on a hamburger bun. (But here you won't miss it.)

PREP TIME: 15 minutes, plus 30 minutes soaking time

COOK TIME: 30 minutes

2 large sweet potatoes, peeled and cut into fries, then soaked in water for 30 minutes and patted dry

2 tablespoons olive oil, plus more for coating

Salt

Freshly ground black pepper

2 garlic cloves, finely chopped

1 small yellow onion, chopped

2 bell peppers, any color, cored and chopped

1 pound ground chicken

1½ tablespoons regular or gluten-free chili powder

1 teaspoon ground cumin

1 (15-ounce) can diced tomatoes, with juice

1 cup water

1. Preheat the oven to 425°F. Line a baking sheet with parchment paper.

2. On the prepared baking sheet, spread out the sweet potatoes and drizzle with some of the olive oil, tossing to coat. Season with salt and pepper.

3. Bake for about 25 minutes, or until crispy, turning once about halfway through the baking time.

4. While the sweet potatoes bake, in a medium pot over medium heat, heat the 2 tablespoons olive oil. Add the garlic, onion, and bell peppers. Cook for about 7 minutes, stirring, until softened.

5. Increase the heat to medium-high and stir in the ground chicken, breaking it up with the spoon. Cook for about 4 minutes, until cooked through and no longer pink.

136

6. Stir in the chili powder, cumin, and 1 teaspoon salt. Add the tomatoes and water. Bring the mixture to a boil. Reduce the heat to low, cover the pan, and simmer for 15 minutes.

STORAGE: Let cool, then store the sweet potato fries and sloppy joe mix separately, each divided among 4 medium resealable containers. Cover, label, and refrigerate for up to 5 days.

REHEAT FROM THE FRIDGE: Remove the fries from the refrigerator and let them sit for 15 minutes. Put 2 paper towels on a microwave-safe plate. Place the fries on the paper towels, spreading them out in an even layer. Drizzle lightly with olive oil. Microwave on high power in 20-second intervals until you've reached your desired temperature. To reheat the sloppy joe, place it in a microwave-safe container, cover with a microwave-safe lid set askew, and microwave on high power for about 3 minutes or until warmed through. To serve, arrange the sweet potato fries on a plate and top with the sloppy joe.

INGREDIENT TIP: Soaking the sweet potatoes in water before oven-frying draws out the excess starch, making the fries extra crispy.

MIX IT UP: Spice things up by stirring some chipotle paste, to suit your taste, into the sloppy joe mix.

Per Serving: Calories: 334; Total fat: 17g; Carbohydrates: 26g; Cholesterol: 90mg; Fiber: 6g; Protein: 23g; Sugar: 10g

Mushroom Veggie Burgers

Makes 4 burgers

These burgers may be vegan, but they're definitely beefy in flavor and texture. What's my inspiration? Amy's Organic Chicago Burgers, which are no longer available. I decided to re-create them, and now I make a double batch and keep them in my freezer for fast, easy lunches or dinners.

PREP TIME: 15 minutes

COOK TIME: 25 minutes

2 tablespoons olive oil, divided

½ small onion, finely chopped

1 (10-ounce) package button mushrooms, stemmed and finely chopped

1 carrot, finely chopped

1 celery stalk, finely chopped

1 cup cooked brown rice

½ cup regular old-fashioned rolled oats or certified gluten-free oats

½ cup chopped walnuts

2 tablespoons all-purpose or gluten-free flour

½ teaspoon salt

1 tablespoon water, plus more as needed

4 regular or gluten-free hamburger buns

4 tomato slices

4 romaine lettuce leaves

Mayonnaise, for serving

1. In a large pan over medium heat, heat 1 tablespoon of the olive oil. Add the onion and cook for about 5 minutes, until softened.

2. Add the mushrooms, carrot, and celery. Cook for about 10 minutes, until the liquid from the mushrooms has evaporated. Transfer to a large bowl and let cool.

3. Stir the brown rice, oats, walnuts, flour, and salt into the cooled veggies. Transfer to a food processor and pulse until coarsely combined. Add the water, 1 tablespoon at a time and up to 1 cup, to achieve a consistency that holds together when pressed. Shape the mixture into 4 patties.

4. In a large skillet over medium-high heat, heat the remaining tablespoon olive oil. Add the patties and cook for about 4 minutes per side, until golden.

138

STORAGE: Store the burgers in each of 4 small resealable containers. Cover, label, and refrigerate for up to 5 days. Place the hamburger buns in resealable sandwich bags, and put the tomato slices and romaine lettuce in each of 4 separate resealable bags. Seal, label, and refrigerate for up to 5 days.

REHEAT FROM THE FRIDGE: Split and toast the bun, if desired. Arrange the burger in a microwave-safe dish and microwave on high power for up to 2 minutes, turning half-way through the cooking time. To serve, spread the bun with some mayonnaise and top the bottom bun with a burger, a tomato slice, a romaine leaf, and the bun top.

Per Serving (1 burger): Calories: 923; Total fat: 22g; Carbohydrates: 72g; Cholesterol: 1mg; Fiber: 11g; Protein: 17g; Sugar: 5g

139

Quinoa Tabbouleh with Hummus

Makes 4 servings

I love to add extra flavor to this dish with one of my favorite spices, za'atar, a traditional eastern Mediterranean intensely aromatic spice blend made with dried herbs such as marjoram or thyme, along with sumac and sesame seeds, which I sprinkle over the hummus before serving. If za'atar isn't available, use your favorite dried herb blend, such as herbes de Provence or Italian seasoning.

PREP TIME: 15 minutes

COOK TIME: 15 minutes

FOR THE TABBOULEH

½ cup quinoa, rinsed well and drained
⅔ cup plus 2 tablespoons water
Salt
½ cucumber, chopped
½ tomato, chopped
Juice of ½ lemon
1 tablespoon olive oil
¼ cup chopped fresh mint leaves
¼ cup chopped fresh parsley
Freshly ground black pepper

FOR THE HUMMUS

1 (15-ounce) can regular or gluten-free
   chickpeas, rinsed and drained
¼ cup tahini, stirred well
1 garlic clove, peeled
2 tablespoons olive oil
Juice of 2 lemons (about ¼ cup)
2 tablespoons water
Salt
Za'atar, for seasoning (optional)

TO MAKE THE TABBOULEH

1. In a large saucepan over high heat, combine the quinoa and water and bring to a boil. Cover the pan, reduce the heat to low, and simmer for about 15 minutes, until all the water is evaporated. Fluff with a fork and season with salt.

2. While the quinoa cooks, in a medium bowl, toss together the cucumber, tomato, lemon juice, olive oil, mint, and parsley. Season with salt and pepper.

TO MAKE THE HUMMUS

3. In a blender or food processor, combine the chickpeas, tahini, garlic, olive oil, lemon juice, and water. Process until creamy but still a bit chunky, about 2 minutes. Taste and season with salt.

140

STORAGE: Evenly divide the tabbouleh among 4 medium resealable containers and the hummus among 4 small resealable containers. Sprinkle the hummus with za'atar (if using). Cover, label, and refrigerate for up to 5 days.

TO SERVE: Place the tabbouleh in a serving bowl and top with the hummus.

INGREDIENT TIP: Use couscous in place of the quinoa to make a classic tabbouleh.

Per Serving: Calories: 380; Total fat: 21g; Carbohydrates: 40g; Cholesterol: 0mg; Fiber: 8g; Protein: 11g; Sugar: 1g

141

Spicy Sichuan Beef with Mixed Vegetables
Makes 4 servings

For this dish, I borrow heat from Indonesia in the form of sambal oelek, a spicy raw chile paste simply made with ground red chiles, vinegar, and salt—which you can find in the international aisle of your local supermarket. Otherwise, substitute sriracha or your favorite hot sauce.

PREP TIME: 10 minutes

COOK TIME: 15 minutes

2 tablespoons olive oil, divided
1 pound beef stir-fry strips
2 tablespoons sambal oelek, or to taste
1 tablespoon tamari
1 tablespoon rice vinegar
1 teaspoon sugar
½ teaspoon Chinese five-spice powder
4 red or green shishito chiles
2 red or green jalapeños, stemmed, seeded (if desired), and thinly sliced
2 celery stalks, thinly sliced
1 carrot, thinly sliced
1 scallion, green and white parts chopped
1 garlic clove, finely chopped
Salt

1. In a large skillet over medium-high heat, heat 1 tablespoon of the olive oil. Add the beef and cook for about 10 minutes, stirring occasionally, until browned. Transfer to paper towels to drain.

2. In a medium bowl, stir together the sambal oelek, tamari, vinegar, sugar, and five-spice powder.

3. Using the same large skillet over high heat, heat the remaining tablespoon olive oil. Add the shishito chiles, jalapeños, celery, carrot, scallion, and garlic. Cook for about 1 minute, stirring constantly, until lightly charred.

4. Stir in the beef and sambal oelek mixture. Cook for 1 minute. Taste and season with salt.

STORAGE: Let cool, then evenly divide the beef mixture among 4 medium resealable containers. Cover, label, and refrigerate for up to 5 days.

REHEAT FROM THE FRIDGE: Transfer the beef to a microwave-safe dish, add 1 tablespoon water, and cover with a paper towel. Microwave on high power for about 2 minutes, until warmed through.

Per Serving: Calories: 238; Total fat: 10g; Carbohydrates: 10g; Cholesterol: 76mg; Fiber: 2g; Protein: 28g; Sugar: 6g

142

Chicken Pasta with Creamy Vodka Sauce

Makes 4 servings

In Italy, I've never seen chicken served in a pasta dish. That said, vodka sauce is more American than it is Italian, and this completely satisfying and easy meal comes together quickly. I'd say that's amore. If you'd prefer not to use vodka, replace it with gluten-free chicken broth or water.

PREP TIME: 15 minutes

COOK TIME: 20 minutes

Salt

1 (8-ounce) box gluten-free penne pasta

2 tablespoons olive oil

1 small onion, finely chopped (about 1 cup)

2 garlic cloves, smashed

½ teaspoon red pepper flakes

2 boneless, skinless chicken breasts (about 8 ounces), cut into strips

½ cup vodka

1 (28-ounce) can tomato purée or crushed tomatoes

1 cup cashew cream (see Cashew Milk tip, page 94) or store-bought dairy-free heavy cream

Freshly ground black pepper

Grated Parmesan Cheese (page 99) or store-bought dairy-free parmesan-style cheese

1. Bring a large pot of salted water to a boil over high heat. Add the pasta and cook for about 10 minutes, until al dente. Drain well.

2. In a medium saucepan over medium heat, heat the olive oil. Add the onion, garlic, and red pepper flakes. Cook for about 4 minutes, stirring occasionally, until the onion is golden.

3. Add the chicken and cook for about 5 minutes, until browned.

4. Stir in the vodka and bring to a boil. Reduce the heat to low and simmer for 2 minutes.

5. Add the tomato purée and cream. Increase the heat to bring to a boil, then reduce the heat to low and simmer for 5 minutes. Taste and season with salt and pepper. Add the pasta and toss to combine.

143

Continues →

STORAGE: Let cool, then evenly divide the pasta among 4 medium resealable containers. Cover, label, and refrigerate for up to 3 days. Evenly divide the parmesan, as desired, into 4 small resealable bags; seal, label, and refrigerate for up to 3 days.

REHEAT FROM THE FRIDGE: Transfer the pasta to a microwave-safe container and add 1 tablespoon water. Cover with a microwave-safe lid set askew, and microwave on high power for 1 minute. Stir. Continue heating in 1-minute increments, adding more water if necessary, until warmed through, about 3 minutes total. Serve topped with the parmesan.

SUBSTITUTION TIP: This recipe can easily be made vegan—just omit the chicken.

Per Serving: Calories: 459; Total fat: 12g; Carbohydrates: 66g; Cholesterol: 44mg; Fiber: 8g; Protein: 23g; Sugar: 13g

Veggie Spaghetti Lo Mein

Makes 4 servings

This stir-fry is hearty enough to be served as a main dish, but it also makes for a great veggie-packed side dish. Either way, there'll be no need to call for Chinese delivery ever again. For this recipe, I use a box of spaghetti from my pantry in place of the more traditional lo mein noodles.

PREP TIME: 10 minutes

COOK TIME: 21 minutes

Salt

1 (16-ounce) box gluten-free spaghetti

½ cup water

¼ cup tamari

2 teaspoons toasted sesame oil

¼ cup avocado oil

1 (8-ounce) package thinly sliced button mushrooms

1 bell pepper, any color, seeded and thinly sliced lengthwise

1 tablespoon finely chopped peeled fresh ginger

2 garlic cloves, finely chopped

6 ounces snow peas, trimmed

3 scallions, green and white parts finely chopped

1. Bring a large pot of salted water to a boil over high heat. Add the spaghetti and cook for about 8 minutes, until al dente. Drain and rinse.

2. In a small bowl, whisk the water, tamari, and sesame oil to blend well.

3. In a large nonstick skillet over high heat, heat the avocado oil. Add the mushrooms and bell pepper. Cook for about 5 minutes, stirring occasionally, until tender and golden.

4. Add the ginger and garlic and cook for 1 minute more.

5. Add the spaghetti and the snow peas and cook for about 2 minutes, stirring occasionally, until the snow peas are just tender. Stir in the tamari mixture and the scallions. Cook for about 5 minutes more, stirring occasionally, until the tamari mixture is absorbed.

145

Continues →

STORAGE: Let cool, then evenly divide the lo mein among 4 medium resealable containers. Cover, label, and refrigerate for up to 5 days.

REHEAT FROM THE FRIDGE: Transfer the lo mein to a microwave-safe container and add 1 tablespoon water. Cover with a microwave-safe lid set askew and microwave on high power for 1 minute. Stir. Continue heating in 1-minute increments, adding more water if necessary, until warmed through, about 3 minutes total.

MIX IT UP: If you'd prefer more protein, chicken, pork, thinly sliced beef, or even shrimp complement the dish nicely.

Per Serving: Calories: 410; Total fat: 18g; Carbohydrates: 50g; Cholesterol: 0mg; Fiber: 8g; Protein: 13g; Sugar: 6g

146

Turmeric-Pistachio Pilaf with Spicy Italian Sausage

Makes 4 servings

This fragrant, vibrantly colored dish is on regular rotation in my house. In the winter months, I like to top the finished dish with a scattering of pomegranate seeds to add a tart crunch that contrasts with the spicy, nutty flavors.

PREP TIME: 15 minutes

COOK TIME: 1 hour, 15 minutes

⅓ cup green lentils

2¾ cups water, divided

1 tablespoon olive oil

1 carrot, finely chopped

1 celery stalk, finely chopped

½ onion, chopped

4 ounces spicy or sweet Italian sausage, casings removed

1 cup brown basmati rice

½ cup shelled raw unsalted pistachios, coarsely chopped

1 teaspoon salt

1 teaspoon ground turmeric

1 teaspoon fennel seeds

2 thyme sprigs

1. In a small saucepan over high heat, combine the lentils and 1 cup of the water. Bring to a boil. Reduce the heat to low and simmer for about 20 minutes, until the lentils are fork-tender.

2. Meanwhile, in a large pot over medium heat, heat the olive oil. Add the carrot, celery, and onion. Cook for about 10 minutes, until the onion is tender.

3. Add the sausage and cook for about 8 minutes, breaking up any clumps, until lightly browned.

4. Stir in the rice, pistachios, salt, turmeric, fennel seeds, and thyme. Cook for about 3 minutes, until the rice is opaque.

147

Continues →

5. Add the cooked lentils and remaining 1¾ cups water and bring to a boil. Cover the pot, reduce the heat to low, and simmer for about 40 minutes, until cooked. Remove from the heat and let steam for 10 minutes. Fluff with a fork.

STORAGE: Let cool, then evenly divide the pilaf among 4 medium resealable containers. Cover, label, and refrigerate for up to 5 days.

REHEAT FROM THE FRIDGE: Transfer the pilaf to a microwave-safe container and add 2 tablespoons water. Cover with a damp paper towel or a microwave-safe lid set askew, and heat on high power for 2 minutes.

MAKE IT EASIER: To speed things up, use white basmati rice and cut the rice cooking time to 15 minutes.

Per Serving: Calories: 376; Total fat: 12g; Carbohydrates: 53g; Cholesterol: 13mg; Fiber: 8g; Protein: 15g; Sugar: 3g

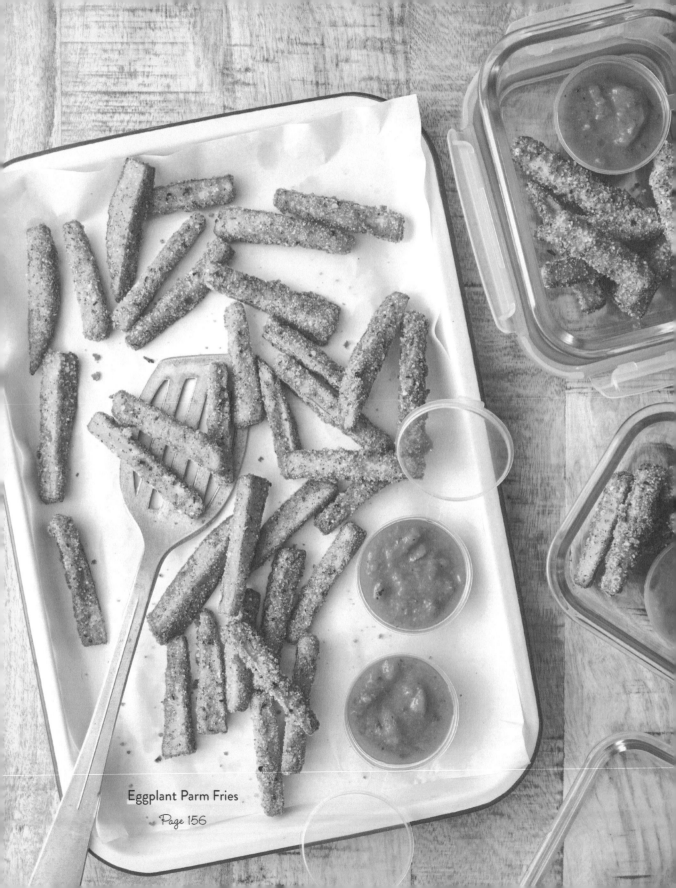

Eggplant Parm Fries

Page 156

SIDES AND SNACKS

※ ※ ※

151

Veggie Fried Cauliflower Rice

Makes 4 servings

No matter the season, this recipe works well served warm or cold.
Using riced cauliflower makes this dish lighter and easier to digest.
Of course, you can also swap in 1 cup of your favorite rice; just cook
it according to the package directions.

PREP TIME: 15 minutes

COOK TIME: 30 minutes

2 tablespoons tamari

2 teaspoons gluten-free hoisin sauce

2¼ teaspoons rice wine vinegar

1½ teaspoons toasted sesame oil

⅛ teaspoon sugar (optional)

1 head cauliflower, stemmed and roughly
   chopped (about 4 cups)

3 tablespoons olive oil, divided

1 tablespoon water

2 large eggs, lightly beaten

Salt

Freshly ground black pepper

3 scallions, green and white parts sliced

1 small onion, finely chopped

1 carrot, finely chopped

½ cup frozen peas, thawed

1. In a small bowl, whisk the tamari, hoisin sauce, vinegar, sesame oil, and sugar (if using) to blend.

2. In a food processor, pulse the cauliflower until finely chopped into a rice-like texture.

3. In a large skillet over medium-high heat, heat 1 tablespoon of the olive oil until hot, but not smoking. Add the cauliflower and cook, stirring often, for about 3 minutes. Add the water, cover the skillet, and cook for about 3 minutes, until softened. Transfer to a plate. Wipe out the skillet with a paper towel.

4. Return the skillet to the stovetop and increase the heat to high. Add 1 tablespoon of the olive oil and heat until hot, but not smoking. Add the eggs and season with salt and pepper. Scramble the eggs for about 1 minute, until fluffy and just cooked through. Transfer to a plate. Wipe out the skillet with a paper towel.

5. Return the skillet to the stovetop and adjust the heat to medium. Add the remaining 1 tablespoon olive oil. Add the scallions, onion, and carrot. Cook for about 4 minutes, stirring, until softened.

6. Fold in the cauliflower and cook for about 10 minutes, until lightly browned.

7. Return the egg to the skillet along with the peas and tamari sauce. Toss everything together and cook for about 3 minutes to heat through.

STORAGE: Evenly divide the fried rice among 4 small resealable containers, cover, label, and refrigerate for up to 5 days.

REHEAT FROM THE FRIDGE: Place the rice in a microwave-safe container and add 2 tablespoons water. Cover with a damp paper towel or a microwave-safe lid set askew, and microwave on high power for 2 minutes.

SUBSTITUTION TIP: To make this vegan, omit the eggs.

Per Serving: Calories: 204; Total fat: 3g; Carbohydrates: 13g; Cholesterol: 93mg; Fiber: 4g; Protein: 7g; Sugar: 6g

French Onion Dip–Stuffed Mushrooms

Makes 12 stuffed mushrooms

Sweet, salty, and deeply umami, these caramelized mushrooms stuffed with onion dip make a satisfying side or appetizer for entertaining. A touch of tamari in the filling adds a wonderfully meaty flavor to the dish.

PREP TIME: 15 minutes

COOK TIME: 40 minutes

1 tablespoon olive oil

1 large red onion, quartered and thinly sliced

1 garlic clove, finely chopped

Salt

Freshly ground black pepper

¼ cup Dairy-Free Sour Cream (page 102) or store-bought dairy-free sour cream

½ teaspoon tamari

1 tablespoon water (optional)

12 large button mushrooms (about 1 pound), stemmed

½ cup crushed gluten-free rice cereal

1. Preheat the oven to 400°F. Line a baking sheet with parchment paper.

2. In a large skillet over medium-high heat, heat the olive oil until hot. Add the red onion, garlic, ¼ teaspoon salt, and ⅛ teaspoon pepper. Cook for about 10 minutes, stirring occasionally, until the onion is softened. Reduce the heat to medium-low and cook until golden, about 10 minutes more.

3. Transfer ¼ cup of the caramelized onion to a blender. Add the sour cream and tamari and blend until smooth. If needed, blend in the water for a thinner dip consistency. Transfer to a bowl. Stir in another ¼ cup of the caramelized onion and season with salt and pepper.

4. Arrange the mushroom caps on the prepared baking sheet, stem-side down.

154

5. Bake for 10 minutes. Flip the mushroom caps over, draining any liquid, and mound some of the onion dip into each one. Sprinkle evenly with the cereal crumbs. Bake for about 20 minutes more, until the mushrooms are tender and the tops are golden.

STORAGE: Let cool, then place 3 stuffed mushrooms in each of 4 medium resealable containers. Cover, label, and refrigerate for up to 3 days. Evenly divide the remaining caramelized onion among 4 small resealable containers. Cover, label, and refrigerate for up to 3 days.

REHEAT FROM THE FRIDGE: Let the stuffed mushrooms and caramelized onion come to room temperature. Transfer the mushrooms to an oven-safe container and top with the caramelized onion. Warm, uncovered, in a 350°F oven or toaster oven for about 15 minutes or until heated through. To reheat in a microwave, place the mushrooms on a microwave-safe dish and top with the caramelized onion. Cover with a damp paper towel. Microwave in 30-second intervals on medium power until sufficiently warmed through.

SUBSTITUTION TIP: You can also use 4 portobello mushrooms in place of the large button mushrooms.

Per Serving (3 mushrooms) Calories: 108; Total fat: 7g; Carbohydrates: 10g; Cholesterol: 0mg; Fiber: 2g; Protein: 5g; Sugar: 5g

Eggplant Parm Fries

Makes 4 servings

Nontraditional, but equally sinful as the standard favorite. That pretty much sums up this vegetable-based parm dish, where I swap eggplant for the classic chicken or veal and bake it instead of fry it. If you don't love spicy food, omit the red pepper flakes in the bread crumb coating.

PREP TIME: 15 minutes

COOK TIME: 20 minutes

Nonstick cooking spray

1 eggplant (about 10 ounces)

1 cup crushed gluten-free rice cereal

¼ cup Grated Parmesan Cheese (page 99) or store-bought dairy-free parmesan-style cheese

2 teaspoons dried parsley flakes

1 teaspoon red pepper flakes

½ teaspoon garlic powder

½ teaspoon salt

½ teaspoon freshly ground black pepper

1 large egg

½ cup canned or jarred marinara sauce, for serving

Olive oil, for serving

1. Preheat the oven to 450°F. Line a baking sheet with parchment paper and lightly coat it with cooking spray.

2. Peel the eggplant, then cut it lengthwise into ¼-inch-thick slices. Cut the slices into sticks about 3 inches long and ¼ inch thick.

3. On a rimmed plate, stir together the cereal crumbs, parmesan, parsley flakes, red pepper flakes, garlic powder, salt, and pepper. On another rimmed plate, whisk the egg.

4. Coat the eggplant strips in the egg, then roll in the crumb mixture to coat well. Place the coated fries on the prepared baking sheet and spray lightly with cooking spray.

5. Bake for about 20 minutes, turning once about halfway through the cooking time, until crisp and golden.

156

STORAGE: Evenly divide the eggplant fries among 4 small resealable containers. Cover, label, and refrigerate for up to 3 days. Evenly divide the marinara sauce among 4 small resealable containers. Cover, label, and refrigerate for up to 5 days.

REHEAT FROM THE FRIDGE: Let the fries come to room temperature. Place 2 paper towels on a microwave-safe plate. Place the fries on the paper towels, spreading them in an even layer. Drizzle lightly with some olive oil. Microwave the fries in 30-second intervals on high power until warmed through. To reheat the marinara, place it in a microwave-safe container, cover with a microwave-safe lid set askew, and heat on high power for about 2 minutes, until warmed through. Serve the fries with the warmed marinara for dipping.

MIX IT UP: For a bit of indulgence, fry the fries instead of baking them. In a large skillet over medium-high heat, heat ½ cup avocado oil until hot. Working in 4 batches and adding ¼ cup oil between batches, cook the eggplant fries for about 2 minutes per side, until golden brown and cooked through.

Per Serving: Calories: 90; Total fat: 4g; Carbohydrates: 9g; Cholesterol: 52mg; Fiber: 3g; Protein: 5g; Sugar: 4g

157

Buffalo Sweet Potato Wedges
Makes 4 servings

Once I realized I could buy dairy-free buffalo wing sauce at my local grocery, my cooking options expanded exponentially. Here, I toss the sauce with potatoes, then roast them for a spicy, crunchy hit of flavor—perfect for dipping into the cool cucumber yogurt–based dipping sauce.

PREP TIME: 10 minutes

COOK TIME: 20 minutes

2 tablespoons dairy-free buffalo
   wing sauce
2 tablespoons avocado oil, plus more
   for serving
1½ pounds sweet potatoes (about
   3 medium), cut into wedges
Salt
1 scallion, green and white parts chopped
1 cup plain dairy-free yogurt
¼ cup chopped cucumber
2 tablespoons chopped fresh parsley
1 tablespoon water, plus more as needed
Freshly ground black pepper
Celery sticks, for serving

1. Preheat the oven to 450°F. Line a baking sheet with parchment paper. Set aside.

2. In a large bowl, whisk the wing sauce and 2 tablespoons avocado oil to combine. Add the sweet potatoes to the bowl and toss to coat. Place the sweet potatoes on the prepared baking sheet and brush with more of the wing sauce from the bowl.

3. Roast for 15 to 20 minutes, turning and brushing once about halfway through the roasting time, until tender. Season with salt, if needed, and sprinkle with the scallion.

4. Meanwhile, in a small bowl, stir together the yogurt, cucumber, and parsley, adding water, 1 tablespoon at a time, to reach your desired consistency. Taste and season with salt and pepper.

158

STORAGE: Dive the buffalo sweet potatoes into 4 portions and place each portion in a medium resealable container. Cover, label, and refrigerate for 3 to 5 days. Divide the sauce among 4 small resealable containers. Cover, label, and refrigerate for up to 5 days.

REHEAT FROM THE FRIDGE: Remove the sweet potato wedges from the fridge and let sit for 15 minutes. Put 2 paper towels on a microwave-safe plate. Place the wedges on the paper towels, spreading them in an even layer. Drizzle lightly with a little avocado oil. Microwave on high power in 20-second intervals until they are sufficiently heated. Serve the wedges with the dipping sauce and some celery sticks.

SUBSTITUTION TIP: Not a sweet potato fan? Swap in Yukon Gold or russet potatoes instead.

Per Serving: Calories: 262; Total fat: 9g; Carbohydrates: 44g; Cholesterol: 0mg; Fiber: 4g; Protein: 3g; Sugar: 32g

Sticky Sesame Chicken Wings
Makes 24 wings

By far, my most ordered dish at Chinese restaurants is sesame chicken. This recipe is a lighter version of that, without all the heavy coating. These wings were a Super Bowl standard at my house for years—they're that good! Now we enjoy them any day of the week.

PREP TIME: 20 minutes

COOK TIME: 30 minutes

24 chicken wings, separated at the joint, wing tips discarded

1 tablespoon olive oil

1 teaspoon salt

½ teaspoon freshly ground black pepper

3 tablespoons tamari

3 tablespoons honey

2 tablespoons rice wine vinegar

2 teaspoons toasted sesame oil

2 garlic cloves, finely chopped

1 scallion, white and green parts finely chopped

1 (1-inch) piece fresh ginger, peeled and finely chopped

Sesame seeds, toasted, for sprinkling

1. Preheat the oven to 450°F. Line a baking sheet with aluminum foil.

2. In a large bowl, toss together the chicken wings, olive oil, salt, and pepper. Place the chicken on the prepared baking sheet.

3. Roast for 15 minutes.

4. Meanwhile, in another large bowl, whisk the tamari, honey, vinegar, sesame oil, garlic, scallion, and ginger until combined. Transfer the partially cooked wings to the sauce and stir to coat. Discard the foil and line the same baking sheet with parchment paper. Place the wings on the prepared baking sheet and roast for 8 minutes.

5. Sprinkle with the sesame seeds and roast for about 5 minutes more, until nicely browned.

160

STORAGE: Let cool, then place 6 wings in each of 4 resealable containers. Cover, label, and refrigerate for up to 3 days.

REHEAT FROM THE FRIDGE: Place 2 paper towels on a microwave-safe plate and top with the wings, then add 2 damp paper towels on top. Microwave in 1-minute intervals on medium power for about 2 minutes, until warmed through.

SUBSTITUTION TIP: Don't have rice vinegar on hand? Use apple cider vinegar instead.

Per Serving (6 wings): Calories: 615; Total fat: 42g; Carbohydrates: 15g; Cholesterol: 170mg; Fiber: 0g; Protein: 44g; Sugar: 13g

Spicy Thai Veggie Rice

Makes 4 servings

The aroma of this spicy rice while it cooks brings my hungry daughter into the kitchen every time. When I want to make this rice dish a more substantial part of our meal, I pan-fry some firm tofu in a bit of hot oil and mix it in.

PREP TIME: 10 minutes

COOK TIME: 25 minutes

1 tablespoon plus 1 teaspoon olive oil, divided

½ cup basmati rice

Grated zest of ½ lime

¾ cup water

½ scallion, white part chopped

Juice of ½ lime

1½ teaspoons red pepper flakes

½ cup sugar

¼ cup rice vinegar

¼ teaspoon salt

6 garlic cloves, finely chopped

½ carrot, cut into rounds

1 cup fresh or frozen broccoli florets

162

STORAGE: Evenly divide the rice among 4 resealable containers. Cover, label, and refrigerate for up to 5 days.

REHEAT FROM THE FRIDGE: Place the rice in a microwave-safe container and add 2 tablespoons water. Cover with a damp paper towel or a microwave-safe lid set askew, and heat on high power for 2 minutes.

INGREDIENT TIP: Want more heat? Add sriracha to taste.

1. In a saucepan over medium heat, heat the 1 teaspoon olive oil. Stir in the rice and toast for 1 minute. Add the lime zest and water and bring to a boil. Reduce the heat to low, cover the pan, and simmer for 15 minutes. Stir in the scallion and lime juice. Fluff the rice with a fork.

2. Meanwhile, in a dry skillet over high heat, toast the red pepper flakes for about 1 minute until fragrant. Add the sugar, vinegar, and salt. Reduce the heat to medium-low and cook for about 5 minutes, until the sugar dissolves. Stir in the garlic. Transfer the sweet and sour sauce to a bowl and let cool.

3. Return the skillet to the stovetop and turn the heat to medium. Add the remaining 1 tablespoon olive oil, the carrot, and broccoli. Cook for about 5 minutes, until the broccoli is tender.

4. Season with the sweet and sour sauce to taste, then toss with the scallion-lime rice.

Per Serving: Calories: 249; Total fat: 5g; Carbohydrates: 48g; Cholesterol: 0mg; Fiber: 1g; Protein: 3g; Sugar: 26g

Loaded Deviled Eggs with Bacon and Chives
Makes 16 egg halves

Sometimes I get fancy and fill a pastry bag with the creamy egg-yolk mixture so I can decoratively pipe it into the egg-white halves. But you don't have to do that. These deviled eggs will be delicious any way you do it. For a hint of heat, serve the deviled eggs with a dash of hot sauce.

PREP TIME: 15 minutes

COOK TIME: 15 minutes

Salt

8 large eggs

3 tablespoons mayonnaise

2 teaspoons Dijon mustard

2 bacon slices, cooked until crisp, then crumbled

2 tablespoons finely chopped celery

2 tablespoons finely chopped scallion

2 teaspoons chopped fresh parsley, plus more for topping

Freshly ground black pepper

STORAGE: Divide the 16 filled egg halves among 4 resealable containers (4 halves per container). Cover, label, and refrigerate for up to 3 days.

COOKING TIP: For a fancy presentation, use a pastry bag fitted with a star tip to pipe the egg-yolk filling into the whites.

Per Serving (4 egg halves): Calories: 241; Total fat: 18g; Carbohydrates: 4g; Cholesterol: 385mg; Fiber: 0g; Protein: 16g; Sugar: 2g

1. Have ready a bowl of ice water.

2. Bring a medium pot of salted water to a boil over high heat. Carefully add the eggs to the pot. Reduce the heat to low and cook for 10 minutes. Drain and transfer the eggs to the ice water. Let cool, then peel.

3. In a medium bowl, whisk the mayonnaise, mustard, three-fourths of the bacon, the celery, scallion, and parsley. Season with salt and pepper.

4. Halve the eggs lengthwise and scoop the yolks into the mayonnaise mixture. Using a fork, mash to combine until creamy. Taste and season with more salt and pepper if needed. Fill each egg half with some of the deviled egg mixture and top with a sprinkle of the remaining bacon and some parsley.

163

Spinach-Tahini Dip with Toasted Pita

Makes 4 servings

I'm a veteran of making spinach-artichoke dips, and this recipe is what happens when I want to put a fresh twist on a family favorite. I've taken out the artichokes and swapped in tahini for the classic cream cheese, sour cream, and sometimes the mayonnaise base. You can spice things up by stirring in some cumin or za'atar to taste, if you have it on hand.

PREP TIME: 10 minutes

COOK TIME: 10 minutes

3 tablespoons olive oil, divided
½ onion, finely chopped
2 garlic cloves, finely chopped
2 (10-ounce) packages frozen chopped
   spinach, thawed and squeezed dry
½ cup tahini, stirred well
¼ cup freshly squeezed lemon juice
1 tablespoon water, plus more as needed
Salt
Freshly ground black pepper
4 pita breads, or more as needed,
   for serving

1. In a large skillet over medium heat, heat 1 tablespoon of the olive oil. Add the onion and garlic. Cook for 3 minutes.

2. Add the spinach. Cook for about 5 minutes, until tender and wilted. Let cool.

3. In a food processor, combine the spinach, tahini, lemon juice, and remaining 2 tablespoons olive oil. Purée until smooth. Add the water, 1 tablespoon at a time, if needed, and process until creamy. Taste and season with salt and pepper.

STORAGE: Divide the dip among 4 resealable containers. Cover, label, and refrigerate for up to 5 days. Place 1 pita bread in each of 4 resealable bags, seal, label, and refrigerate for up to 5 days.

REHEAT FROM THE FRIDGE: Toast the pitas, cut into triangles, and serve with the dip.

SUBSTITUTION TIP: Make this gluten-free by using a gluten-free variety of pita.

Per Serving: Calories: 478; Total fat: 28g; Carbohydrates: 46g; Cholesterol: 0mg; Fiber: 8g; Protein: 15g; Sugar: 2g

Nutty Pretzel Snack Bars
Makes 6 bars

Do you want to know the best thing about making your own snack bars? You know exactly what ingredients are in them. You also know just how healthy you can make them because, let's be honest, you know what you— or your kids—will eat. With their salty sweetness and addicting crunch, these easy-to-make snack bars are the go-to treats for my kids. If you're gluten-free, use gluten-free oats, rice cereal, and pretzels.

PREP TIME: 10 minutes

COOK TIME: 30 minutes

Nonstick cooking spray

1 cup old-fashioned rolled oats or certified gluten-free oats

1 cup bread crumbs or gluten-free rice cereal

½ cup chopped raw almonds

½ cup chopped raw cashews

½ cup regular pretzel sticks or gluten-free pretzels

⅛ teaspoon salt

½ cup pure maple syrup

⅓ cup creamy almond butter

1. Preheat the oven to 325°F. Coat a 9-by-5 by-3-inch loaf pan with cooking spray and line it with overhanging parchment paper.

2. In a large bowl, toss together the oats, bread crumbs, almonds, cashews, pretzels, and salt.

3. In a small saucepan over low heat, stir together the maple syrup and almond butter. Cook for about 3 minutes, until combined. Pour this over the oat mixture and toss to evenly coat. Transfer the mixture to the prepared loaf pan and, using a piece of parchment coated with cooking spray, press down firmly to spread the mixture evenly in the pan.

4. Bake for 12 minutes. Let cool completely.

Continues →

165

5. Preheat the oven to 250°F. Line a baking sheet with parchment paper and place a wire rack on top.

6. Using the overhanging parchment, remove the bar mixture from the loaf pan. Cut it into 6 bars. Place the bars, gooey-side up, on the wire rack.

7. Bake for about 15 minutes, until almost dry to the touch.

STORAGE: Let cool, then divide the 6 bars among 6 resealable bags. Seal and store at room temperature for up to 5 days.

MIX IT UP: Use your favorite nuts and seeds—like peanuts, pecans, or sunflower seeds—in place of the almonds and cashews.

Per Serving (1 bar): Calories: 421; Total fat: 23g; Carbohydrates: 46g; Cholesterol: 0mg; Fiber: 6g; Protein: 11g; Sugar: 19g

166

Coconut-Pecan Sweet and Salty Bars
Makes 6 bars

This recipe raises the bar (pun intended) on the healthy without skimping on the happy. These snack bars are packed with protein-rich, energy-boosting nuts—just in time for your next on-the-go breakfast or afternoon pick-me-up.

PREP TIME: 10 minutes

COOK TIME: 27 minutes

Nonstick cooking spray
¾ cup sliced raw almonds
¾ cup unsweetened shredded coconut
½ cup coarsely chopped raw pecans
⅓ cup gluten-free rice cereal
¼ cup brown rice syrup
2 tablespoons molasses
¼ teaspoon salt
¼ teaspoon ground cinnamon

STORAGE: Let cool, then divide the 6 bars among 6 resealable bags. Seal and store at room temperature for up to 5 days.

MIX IT UP: Kick up the spice by adding a pumpkin spice blend or add a savory element with a barbecue spice blend in place of the cinnamon.

Per Serving (1 bar): Calories 299, Total fat 22g, Carbohydrates 23g, Cholesterol 0mg, Fiber 5g, Protein 5g, Sugar 14g

1. Preheat the oven to 325°F. Coat a 9-by-5-by-3-inch loaf pan with cooking spray, and line it with overhanging parchment paper.

2. In a large bowl, stir together the almonds, coconut, pecans, cereal crumbs, brown rice syrup, molasses, salt, and cinnamon until combined. Transfer the mixture to the prepared loaf pan and, using a piece of parchment coated with cooking spray, press down firmly to spread the mixture evenly in the pan.

3. Bake for 12 minutes. Let cool completely.

4. Preheat the oven to 250°F. Line a baking sheet with parchment paper and place a wire rack on top.

5. Using the overhanging parchment, remove the bar mixture from the pan. Cut it evenly into 6 bars. Place the bars, gooey-side up, on the wire rack.

6. Bake for about 15 minutes, until almost dry to the touch.

167

Spice-Roasted Rosemary Mixed Nuts

Makes 4 servings

I love playing with the different tastes and textures in every recipe
I develop. These roasted nuts are no exception. I start by tossing nuts
and seeds with curry powder and cinnamon, then sweeten the deal with
a drizzle of maple syrup. Then, I scatter on some chopped fresh rosemary for
a deliciously playful dance of sweet, earthy, woodsy flavors.

PREP TIME: 10 minutes

COOK TIME: 12 minutes

½ cup raw pecans

½ cup raw almonds

½ cup raw cashews

2 tablespoons raw pumpkin seeds

2 tablespoons curry powder

1 teaspoon ground cinnamon

1 teaspoon salt

2 tablespoons pure maple syrup

1 tablespoon avocado oil

1 tablespoon chopped fresh
   rosemary leaves

1. Preheat the oven to 350°F.
   Line a baking sheet with
   parchment paper.

2. In a large bowl, toss together
   the pecans, almonds, cashews,
   pumpkin seeds, curry powder, cinnamon, salt, maple syrup, avocado
   oil, and rosemary to evenly coat
   everything. Spread the mixture
   on the prepared baking sheet in
   an even layer.

3. Bake for 8 to 12 minutes, until
   toasted.

STORAGE: Let cool, then evenly divide
among 4 resealable bags. Seal and store
at room temperature for up to 5 days.

INGREDIENT TIP: If this mixture is
too spicy for you, omit the curry powder
or cinnamon—or both.

Per Serving: Calories: 349; Total fat: 29g; Carbohydrates:
19g; Cholesterol: 0mg; Fiber: 5g; Protein: 8g; Sugar: 8g

168

Pomegranate-Lime Chia Cooler

Makes 4 coolers

I love to drink this cooler as a snack between meals, after workouts, and throughout the summer to keep hydrated. The best part? It's not just refreshing, but also filling.

PREP TIME: 10 minutes

5 cups water
3 cups pomegranate juice
¼ cup freshly squeezed lime juice
½ cup chia seed meal
Salt

In a blender, combine the water, pomegranate juice, lime juice, chia meal, and a pinch of salt. Blend on high speed for 3 minutes.

STORAGE: Refrigerate in 4 resealable containers for at least 2 hours or up to 5 days.

TO SERVE: Shake the contents of 1 refrigerated container well.

INGREDIENT TIP: Can't find ground chia seeds? Use an electric spice grinder or mortar and pestle to crush whole chia seeds into a powder.

169

Per Serving (1 cooler): Calories 252; Total fat 9g; Carbohydrates 41g; Cholesterol 0mg; Fiber 10g; Protein 5g; Sugar 24g

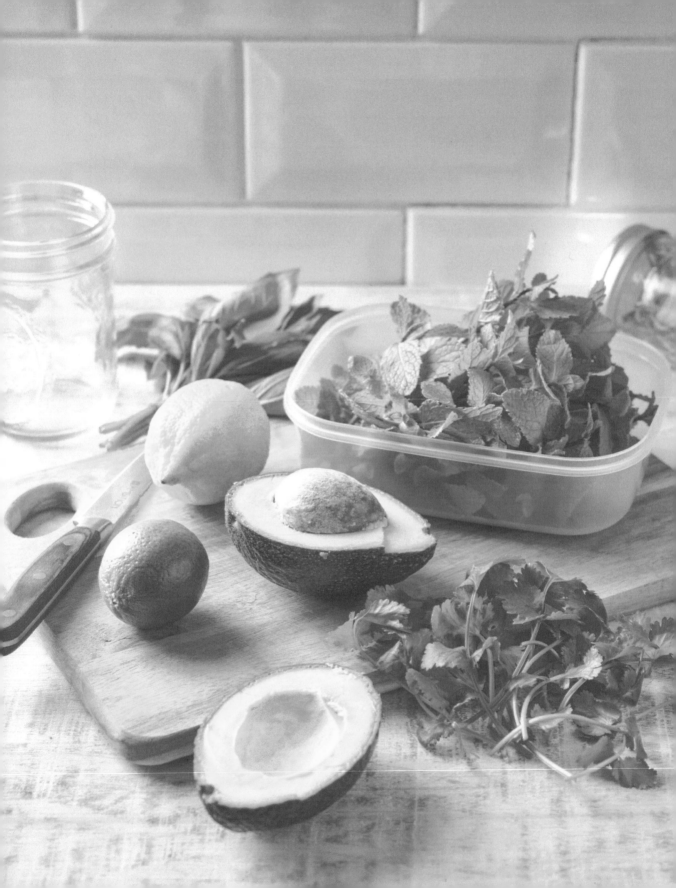

MEASUREMENT CONVERSIONS

VOLUME EQUIVALENTS (LIQUID)

US Standard	US Standard (ounces)	Metric (approximate)
2 tablespoons	1 fl. oz.	30 mL
¼ cup	2 fl. oz.	60 mL
½ cup	4 fl. oz.	120 mL
1 cup	8 fl. oz.	240 mL
1½ cups	12 fl. oz.	355 mL
2 cups or 1 pint	16 fl. oz.	475 mL
4 cups or 1 quart	32 fl. oz.	1 L
1 gallon	128 fl. oz.	4 L

OVEN TEMPERATURES

Fahrenheit (F)	Celsius (C) (approximate)
250°F	120°C
300°F	150°C
325°F	165°C
350°F	180°C
375°F	190°C
400°F	200°C
425°F	220°C
450°F	230°C

VOLUME EQUIVALENTS (DRY)

US Standard	Metric (approximate)
⅛ teaspoon	0.5 mL
¼ teaspoon	1 mL
½ teaspoon	2 mL
¾ teaspoon	4 mL
1 teaspoon	5 mL
1 tablespoon	15 mL
¼ cup	59 mL
⅓ cup	79 mL
½ cup	118 mL
⅔ cup	156 mL
¾ cup	177 mL
1 cup	235 mL
2 cups or 1 pint	475 mL
3 cups	700 mL
4 cups or 1 quart	1 L

WEIGHT EQUIVALENTS

US Standard	Metric (approximate)
½ ounce	15 g
1 ounce	30 g
2 ounces	60 g
4 ounces	115 g
8 ounces	225 g
12 ounces	340 g
16 ounces or 1 pound	455 g

REFERENCES

Fresh N' Lean (blog). *Benefits of Going Dairy-Free.* Accessed February 12, 2020. https://www.freshnlean.com/real-reasons-part-2-going-dairy-free.

Go Dairy Free (blog). *Dairy-Free Benefits: The Top 10 Reasons to Go Dairy-Free.* Accessed February 12, 2020. https://www.godairyfree.org/news/dairy-free-benefits.

Health magazine. "5 Things That Might Happen to Your Body When You Give Up Dairy." Accessed February 12, 2020. https://www.health.com/nutrition/eliminate-dairy-diet.

Nutricia Research. "Allergy, the Immune-Gut Interplay." Accessed February 12, 2020. https://www.nutriciaresearch.com/allergy/allergy-the-immune-gut-interplay.

The/Thirty (blog). *I Gave Up Dairy for 21 Days—Here's What Happened to My Skin and Body.* Accessed February 12, 2020. https://thethirty.whowhatwear.com/benefits-of-dairy-free.

Well + Good. "I Tried Cutting Out Dairy for a Week—Here's What Happens." Accessed February 12, 2020. https://www.wellandgood.com/good-food/what-happens-when-you-cut-dairy.

INDEX

173

174

176

178

180

ABOUT THE AUTHOR

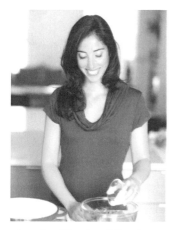

Silvana Nardone is the author of *The 30-Minute Dairy-Free Cookbook, Silvana's Gluten-Free and Dairy-Free Kitchen: Timeless Favorites Transformed,* and *Cooking for Isaiah: Gluten-Free & Dairy-Free Recipes for Easy, Delicious Meals.* She successfully launched Cooking for Isaiah® by Silvana Nardone, a gluten-free, dairy-free flour blend and baking mix company that gives people who are dairy or gluten sensitive the freedom to cook and bake again. Previously, Silvana was the founding editor-in-chief of celebrity chef Rachael Ray's magazine, *Rachael Ray Every Day,* and the owner of an Italian bakery, Fanciulla. She lives in New York City.

CPSIA information can be obtained
at www.ICGtesting.com
Printed in the USA
JSRC032318090620
R10135100001B/R101351PG6104JSX1B/1